PRAISE FOR ISA CHANDRA MOSKOWITZ AND TERRY HOPE ROMERO'S

VEGANOMICON

"The next revolution in neo-vegan cuisine."
—*Philadelphia City Paper*

"Exuberant and unapologetic…the eclectic collection of dishes is a testament to the authors' sincere love of cooking and culinary exploration."
—*Saveur*

"[A] slam-bang effort…making admirable use of every fruit and vegetable under the sun."
—*Publishers Weekly* starred review

"It's full of great food that anyone would love."
—*Baltimore Sun*

"[Moskowitz and Romero] are as …funny when kibbitzing as they are subtle and intuitive when putting together vegan dishes."
—*New York Times Book Review*

"The *Betty Crocker's Cookbook* of the vegan world."
—*Bitch*

VEGAN CUPCAKES TAKE OVER THE WORLD

"Written chattily and supportively for even the most oven-phobic…reading this is like having a couple of fun, socially conscious post-punk pals over for a slumber party… Each page of this cookbook contains an irresistible delight."
—*Bust*

"I can't wait to have a cupcake/champagne party so we can try them all!"
—Alicia Silverstone, author of *The Kind Diet*

Appetite for Reduction

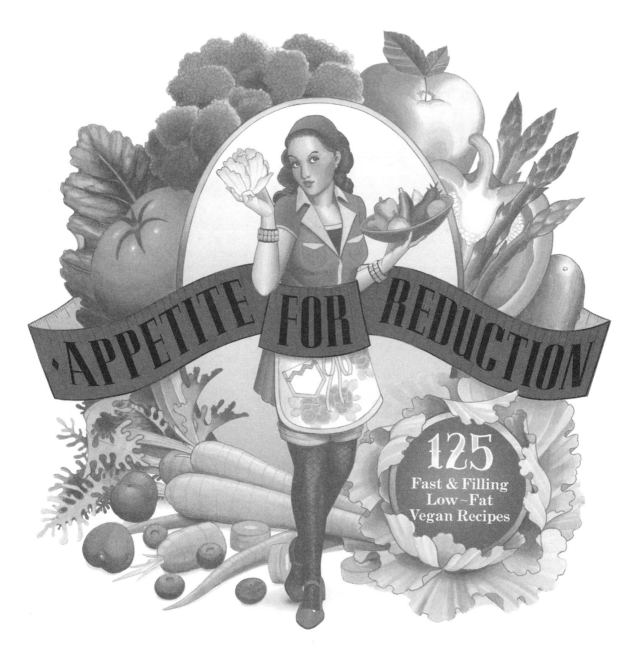

ISA CHANDRA MOSKOWITZ

with Matthew Ruscigno, MPH, RD

Da Capo Lifelong Books   A Member of the Perseus Books Group

Editorial production by Marrathon Production Services. www.marrathon.net
Book design by Lisa Diercks

Cataloging-in-Publication data for this book is available from the Library of Congress.
First Da Capo Press edition 2011
ISBN: 978-1-60094-049-1

Published by Da Capo Press
A Member of the Perseus Books Group
www.dacapopress.com

Note: The information in this book is true and complete to the best of our knowledge. This book is intended only as an informative guide for those wishing to know more about health issues. In no way is this book intended to replace, countermand, or conflict with the advice given to you by your own physician. The ultimate decision concerning care should be made between you and your doctor. We strongly recommend you follow his or her advice. Information in this book is general and is offered with no guarantees on the part of the authors or Da Capo Press. The authors and publisher disclaim all liability in connection with the use of this book.

Da Capo Press books are available at special discounts for bulk purchases in the U.S. by corporations, institutions, and other organizations. For more information, please contact the Special Markets Department at the Perseus Books Group, 2300 Chestnut Street, Suite 200, Philadelphia, PA, 19103, or call (800) 810-4145, ext. 5000, or e-mail special.markets@perseusbooks.com.

2 3 4 5 6 7 8 9

Dedicated To Marlene Stewart.
My Mom and the world's best Grandmo

Contents

CHAPTER 7. SOUL-SATISFYING SOUPS **197**

CHAPTER 8. COMFORT CURRIES, CHILI, & STEWS **225**

Introduction

NOT LOOKING FORWARD TO A TINY FROZEN ENTRÉE FOR dinner? Can't bear the thought of rice cakes and diet shakes? How about a simmering pot of aromatic curry bursting with color, pasta smothered in plenty of creamy pesto, a stick-to-your-ribs chili, crispy onion rings with a juicy center, or a fully loaded lasagna?

This isn't your mother's low-fat cookbook. No foolish tricks, no bizarre concoctions, no chemicals, no frozen meals, no fake anything—this is cooking with real food, with a real budget, and for real life. This is cooking with an *appetite*.

Healthy cooking doesn't have to mean deprivation. It doesn't mean restraint, it doesn't mean willpower, and to hell with the idea of "being good." Utilizing every plant-based food there is and inspired by cooking techniques and traditions from across the globe, I wanted to create a low-calorie, low-fat cookbook brimming with nutritious meals that are satisfying at every level, from your taste buds to your tummy. Because what's the point of filling yourself up on foods that you aren't even enjoying?

To save you the trouble, all of the recipes have been reviewed by a registered dietician, the talented Matt Ruscigno! All of the nutritional info has been calculated, and Matt has made sure that they are in tip-top form. The recipes are all based on pantry-friendly ingredients, and most come in under 400 calories. Some of them are even less than 200. And to sweeten the pot (almost literally), the book was designed with the busy weeknight chef in mind. The ingredients are easy to find and many of the recipes come together in thirty minutes, and the ones that don't will give you plenty of downtime, so that while your dinner is busy cooking away, you can be off finishing your novel, doing your nails, or whatever it is you do in your spare time. A little light carpentry, perhaps?

Why I Wrote this Book

You probably have a few reasons of your own for wanting to cook healthier, and maybe we cover them in **Mission: Nutrition** (page 5).

But I wrote this book for me!

For years I was at a weight I was happy with, but eventually (like most people) I began to pack on the pounds once again. Not that I need a good reason to gain weight, but I do have a few. I wrote a bunch of cookbooks—one dealing completely in cupcakes—and I was constantly surrounded by food. I also quit smoking (best decision I ever made) and found it difficult to keep cookies from hopping into my mouth instead. But on top of that I was diagnosed with two medical issues that are known to make it difficult to lose weight: PCOS (polycystic ovary syndrome, a hormonal issue) and hypothyroidism (an underactive thyroid gland, which regulates metabolism). So even if I wasn't eating more than usual, my slower metabolism would guarantee I put on some extra pounds.

My decision to change my diet wasn't an easy one. I definitely didn't want to perpetuate all the fat-phobia in this country and the systemized berating of big girls. I don't think fat makes you a moral failure, I don't think fat means you're lazy, and I definitely don't believe that the ridiculous beauty standards that our society has created for women are good reasons to change your diet. Your weight is not your worth! And I think women have every right in the world to not worry about what they're eating, not obsess over the scale, and not put up with all the BS that comes our way because of our weight. I believe in health at any size, or heck, even the right *not* to be healthy at any size!

My decision really was a personal one. My knees were achy, my periods were irregular, and my energy levels were low. I needed to change what I was eating—less fat, less sugar—and I needed to get more active. Would that lead to weight loss? I really wasn't sure! There are hundreds of books dedicated to the subject of long term weight loss, and if those tomes don't produce many conclusive answers, I am definitely not about to attempt to do so. What I can tell you is that when I eat low-fat, plant-based meals I feel better, weight does come off, and, unless I skip breakfast or something, I never feel hungry. It's become a sustainable way of life for me! I still enjoy a cupcake now and then, and I still cook and eat more decadently a few times a week. Although I'm sure there are ways to make myself lose weight faster, I am also sure that it would come right back on. Call it a "diet," call it a "lifestyle change," whatever! The most important thing is enjoying food, enjoying life, and doing what makes you feel good, and not just for the moment. (Ice cream is so love-'em-and-leave-'em; I'm looking for something more stable.)

So, yes, I wrote this book for me—but of course I hope that it rocks your stove top, too. Low-fat cookbooks can be a war zone for women. I wanted to create something fun and positive, something that would empower you in the produce aisle and give you a reason to sport that cute vintage apron. I want you to love your kitchen, love yourself, and, yeah, maybe to love tofu just a little bit, too.

With love and raised spatulas,
Isa Chandra Moskowitz

But this book isn't only about reducing fat and calories. Appetite for Reduction also means...

Reducing unhealthy ingredients: Get ready to become the mayor of the produce aisle! When you start cooking with an appetite, the snack product aisle becomes an old flame you can't believe you were ever into. You don't know what you ever saw in those not-even-foods! A whole new world of fun, colorful ingredients will open up to you.

Reducing your environmental impact: We've all heard the term ecological footprint. Well, it's not just black-wearing college students who claim you should give up animal products to save the world. A 2009 United Nations Report states that a shift toward a vegan diet is necessary to save the world from hunger, poverty, and the worst impacts of climate change. The carbon emissions and methane from an animal-based diet are not sustainable for our planet. Switching to a whole-food, plant-based diet will also cut down on the amount of packaging you use. Keep eating those fast-food burgers and there won't be a planet on which you can eat those fast-food burgers! You'll just be floating in space with the burger, I guess.

Reducing your grocery store costs: Just as it's a myth that it takes chewing gum seven years to digest if you swallow it, it's a myth that plant-based diets are more expensive. If you're eating mostly whole foods, you'll see a dramatic drop at the cash register. Beans and grains are cheap as, well, beans! You'll spend a little extra on fresh veggies, especially organic ones, but even an omnivorous diet includes some vegetables. If you're living on packaged store-bought vegan sausages, then, yes, the costs can be high, but this book will help you to get out of that rut!

Reducing animal suffering: I try to avoid images of slaughterhouses and chickens in cages because, hot damn, is it depressing. But check out videos and movies such as *Meet Your Meat* or *Earthlings* and you might lose your taste for meat, too. Even grass-fed cows raised in nice places meet a dismal end, and those free-range chickens are not as free as you may think. I extend the love I have for my kitty cats to the entire animal kingdom. If you've ever seen a baby cow torn away from her mother at just a few months old, you'll understand why this book is not just vegetarian, but vegan, excluding animal products all together.

Increasing your devotion to cruelty-free hairspray and '80s glam rock: If you're not enjoying what you're doing and not enjoying what you're *eating*, you probably aren't going to stick with it. That's the bottom line! *Appetite for Reduction* is all about enjoying it!

Metric Conversions

• The recipes in this book have not been tested with metric measurements, so some variations might occur.

• Remember that the weight of dry ingredients varies according to the volume or density factor: 1 cup of flour weighs far less than 1 cup of sugar, and 1 tablespoon doesn't necessarily hold 3 teaspoons.

GENERAL FORMULA FOR METRIC CONVERSION

Ounces to grams	→	multiply ounces by 28.35
Grams to ounces	→	multiply ounces by 0.035
Pounds to grams	→	multiply pounds by 453.5
Pounds to kilograms	→	multiply pounds by 0.45
Cups to liters	→	multiply cups by 0.24
Fahrenheit to Celsius	→	subtract 32 from Fahrenheit temperature, multiply by 5, divide by 9
Celsius to Fahrenheit	→	multiply Celsius temperature by 9, divide by 5, add 32

LINEAR MEASUREMENTS

½ in	=	1½ cm
1 inch	=	2½ cm
6 inches	=	15 cm
8 inches	=	20 cm
10 inches	=	25 cm
12 inches	=	30 cm
20 inches	=	50 cm

VOLUME (DRY) MEASUREMENTS

¼ teaspoon	=	1 milliliter
½ teaspoon	=	2 milliliters
¾ teaspoon	=	4 milliliters
1 teaspoon	=	5 milliliters
1 tablespoon	=	15 milliliters
¼ cup	=	59 milliliters
⅓ cup	=	79 milliliters
½ cup	=	118 milliliters
⅔ cup	=	158 milliliters
¾ cup	=	177 milliliters
1 cup	=	225 milliliters
4 cups or 1 quart	=	1 liter
½ gallon	=	2 liters
1 gallon	=	4 liters

VOLUME (LIQUID) MEASUREMENTS

1 teaspoon	=	⅙ fluid ounce	=	5 milliliters
1 tablespoon	=	½ fluid ounce	=	15 milliliters
2 tablespoons	=	1 fluid ounce	=	30 milliliters
¼ cup	=	2 fluid ounces	=	60 milliliters
⅓ cup	=	2⅔ fluid ounces	=	79 milliliters
½ cup	=	4 fluid ounces	=	118 milliliters
1 cup or ½ pint	=	8 fluid ounces	=	250 milliliters
2 cups or 1 pint	=	16 fluid ounces	=	500 milliliters
4 cups or 1 quart	=	32 fluid ounces	=	1,000 milliliters
1 gallon	=	4 liters		

OVEN TEMPERATURE EQUIVALENTS, FAHRENHEIT (F) AND CELSIUS (C)

100°F	=	38°C
200°F	=	95°C
250°F	=	120°C
300°F	=	150°C
350°F	=	180°C
400°F	=	205°C
450°F	=	230° C

WEIGHT (MASS) MEASUREMENTS

1 ounce	=	30 grams		
2 ounces	=	55 grams		
3 ounces	=	85 grams		
4 ounces	=	¼ pound	=	125 grams
8 ounces	=	½ pound	=	240 grams
12 ounces	=	¾ pound	=	375 grams
16 ounces	=	1 pound	=	454 grams

Mission: Nutrition

BY MATT RUSCIGNO, MPH, RD

ALL OF ISA'S RECIPES IN THIS BOOK ARE PLANT-BASED, LOW-fat, satisfying, and nutrient-dense: lots of nutrients with fewer calories. We've included the nutrition info so you can see the amount of protein, fiber, iron, calcium, and other key nutrients for each serving. But the beauty is you can follow these recipes and not have to obsess over calories to maintain your weight.

Studies show that vegetarians have lower cholesterol levels and blood pressure and lower rates of type-2 diabetes, hypertension, heart disease, and cancer—the leading causes of death in United States. The reason? A diet low in animal products and higher in fruits, vegetables, whole grains, nuts, and soy products.

CAN YOU REALLY GET YOUR IMPORTANT NUTRIENTS THIS WAY? YES, AND THEN SOME!

Vegan nutrition is different from the standard Western diet whose nutrients tend to come from one major source, such as iron from meat or calcium from dairy. As a vegan, you'll get your nutrition from a bunch of different foods—and this is to your advantage! When smaller amounts of nutrients are eaten at a time, their absorption is actually better. And you are not dependent on just one food. You can get your iron from beans or from whole grains. Avoiding wheat? Eat leafy greens. In fact, variety is crucial when planning your meals, to get all of the nutrients you need. And as mentioned above, fruits and veggies are also nutrient-*dense*, packing a whole lot of benefits for a very small amount of calories. The same is true for whole grains and beans. A win-win scenario!

But good nutrition is also about much more than just, well, nutrients. Back in the day, the experts in the field were chiefly concerned with preventing deficiencies: consuming enough vitamin C so people didn't die of scurvy; getting enough iron to prevent anemia. This is still important, but eventually, some smart folks realized that when you eat a whole food, you're getting even more health benefits beyond the recommended daily allowance of this or that mineral. What researchers have found is that almost all of the foods with these extra benefits come from plants.

For example, only plant foods contain thousands of phytochemicals—such as lycopene in tomatoes, isoflavones in soybeans, flavonoids in tea, and allicin in garlic—which are linked to disease prevention. Plant foods also contain antioxidants, which can help combat cell damage (associated with age-related diseases, cellular diseases such as cancer, and chronic diseases such as heart disease). Good sources are berries, apples, and other fruits; vegetables; chocolate; coffee; and wine. There is no daily recommendation for antioxidants and the best way to get them is directly through whole foods.

Now let's take a look at basic nutrient requirements. These are the ones that are most often asked about in vegan nutrition and we want to be sure you know what you are getting.

"But where do you get your _____ from?"
Anyone reducing meat and dairy consumption has heard this question. A plant-based diet not only has the bases covered, you are also getting more of this good stuff with less fat and cholesterol than you would on an animal product–based diet. Here's a quick rundown.

Protein. Protein is a combination of amino acids, nine of which are essential to human life. Luckily, plants have all of the amino acids you need!

High-protein foods include beans, nuts, seeds, and whole grains such as wheat, quinoa, and millet. In general, aim for 10 to 15 percent of your calories to come from protein. In grams it looks like this: 37 to 56 grams per day on a 1,500-calorie diet; 50 to 75 grams per day on a 2,000-calorie diet. Many of the whole-grain and bean recipes in this book have 10 to 15 percent or more calories from protein per serving.

Proteins (such as those from grains and beans) don't even need to be combined during a meal for you to consume the right amount of amino acids, as it was once believed. You just need to eat enough protein from different foods each day and you'll get your amino acids without a problem. It's also important to remember that even vegetables have protein; for example, kale is 45 percent protein and zucchini is 28 percent protein. You don't need to look any further than the nutrition info provided in these recipes to see where you'll get your protein!

Iron. You need iron every day for your red blood cells to carry oxygen and nutrients to your cells. The well-known deficiency, anemia, has side effects that include fatigue and malaise. No one is happy when he or she is not getting enough iron. Fortunately, iron is found in abundance in plants. Good sources include lentils, soybeans, chickpeas, black beans, collard greens, oatmeal, whole grains, and enriched grains. Plant-based diets tend to be very high in iron and some research[1] shows

---

1. E. H. Haddad, et al., "Dietary Intake and Biochemical, Hematologic and Immune Status Compared with Nonvegetarians" *American Journal of Clinical Nutrition.* 70 (1999): 586S–93S.

that vegans have better iron levels than vegetarians do. Dairy contains zero iron but most plant foods contain at least some.

Just because there is iron in a food doesn't mean that it's bioavailable, meaning your body is able to absorb it. Plant foods contain non-heme iron and, when eaten in combination with vitamin C–rich foods, its absorption can increase sixfold. Think iron-rich beans and rice with vitamin C–rich salsa. Or hummus (whose iron is from chickpeas) and lemon juice (for vitamin C). The tannins in coffee and tea can interfere with iron absorption, so separate your high-iron meals or iron supplement from these beverages by a few hours. And if you think you may be low in iron, get it checked! Low iron levels increase very quickly when higher amounts of iron are eaten.

Calcium. Calcium is the key component in strong bones and teeth, but also has many functions in your blood. It maintains blood pressure, helps in blood clotting, and is essential for muscle contractions such as your heartbeat. When you don't have enough in your blood, it is taken from your bones, which reduces bone density.

Whenever someone eats fewer dairy products, the question of calcium intake arises. Have no fear: Green leafy vegetables such as collards, kale, and bok choy, broccoli, black-eyed peas, fortified nondairy milks, and calcium-set tofu are all good sources. Orange juice with added calcium and other enriched foods are also available. Lastly, calcium supplements or multivitamins that contain calcium can be also used. When supplementing with calcium, make sure you're using tablets with a high percentage of "elemental calcium," which means the amount of bioavailable calcium. Check to see that it says "amino acid–chelated" calcium somewhere on the bottle; your bones will thank you.

Zinc. Needed daily, but only in small amounts, zinc is required for growth, reproduction, a healthy immune system, metabolism, and a number of other functions. Zinc is widely available in whole grains, beans such as lentils and chickpeas, nuts, enriched cereals, and some fake meat products (be sure to check the label).

Vitamin B12. Talking about a vegan diet is like that game where you say a word and the other person says the first thing that comes to mind. "Vegan"—"B12!" It's as if the entire diet hinges on this one vitamin! Vitamin B12 is available in such vegan foods as fortified nondairy milks, cereals, and nutritional yeast, as well as energy bars such as Clif and Luna. B12 deficiency is extremely rare and most often occurs when there are genetic issues affecting absorption or diets restricted far beyond veganism. Not that B12 is unimportant; it is crucial for your brain, nervous system, and red blood cells. You need 2.4 micrograms every day. Please do pay attention and make sure you have a daily source from fortified foods or a sublingual or spray supplement. Just don't let the name association game get you down! If you are unsure, get a lab test to know your B12 levels.

Sodium. Salt is more than just a flavor enhancer! Sodium is a mineral required by your body for a number of functions; for example, sodium is required for water to get through your cell walls. Everyone gets enough as it naturally occurs in plants; the issue is that some people get too much and that is a risk factor for hypertension (high blood pressure). Fortunately, sodium is easy to monitor because you can control how much salt you add while preparing foods. Lower-sodium options exist for soy sauce, vegetable broths, and other prepared foods. If you are watching your sodium, choose these options when working with these recipes.

Say It with Me: High Fiber, Low Fat
Fiber. Fiber is only found in plant foods such as beans, whole grains, vegetables and fruits. It adds bulk to your diet, which fills you up quicker and keeps you full longer—great when watching your weight. It's recommended that you consume 25–35 grams of fiber per day. The dishes in this book will help you reach that goal. Fiber also regulates blood sugar, lowers cholesterol, and reduces your risk for heart disease—an added benefit of these recipes. And fiber helps with weight control even before you eat it. These meals give you a serving with more food and volume, but fewer calories. It's said that we eat with our eyes, and a full plate of fiber-rich foods looks satisfying, not restricting.

The Skinny on Fat. Yes, this book is low fat, but it's not *no* fat. If you remember that diet craze of the '80s, where people ate nothing but sugary cardboard cookies and didn't even lose weight, you'll know that zero-fat diets aren't a good thing. In fact, the truth is your body needs fat. You need it to properly absorb vitamins, you need it to keep your brain functioning, and you need it to keep your body working as it should. Beyond health reasons, fat is a crucial component. Even minimal amounts of fat help you feel satiated. It brings out the flavor of foods and aids cooking by caramelizing and browning.

So you need fat, but not too much fat and not the wrong kinds of fat (such as saturated fat or trans fat). That sounds like a pain in the butt to negotiate, but it's not really as confusing as it sounds. For one thing, most of the unhealthy fats come in the form of animal products. If you're eating little to no animal products, you're more than halfway there. Other kinds of unhealthy fats come from how you process the food—think deep-frying or using chemically processed hydrogenated oils. (Take fast-food French fries, which start with potatoes, then saturated and trans fats are added, 'til half the calories come from fat!) Limit those and you're pretty much left with the good fats.

So why does even good fat sometimes get a bad rap? Because fat has more calories per gram than carbohydrate or protein does. Think about an avocado and an apple that are the same size—the avocado has twice as many calories! Keep this in mind when planning your meals and don't be afraid to have these healthy fats with every meal. You need them!

The handy Big Fat Fat Glossary uses multisyllabic words that get everyone in a tizzy. Don't be fatphobic! Use it to determine just what kind of fats you're dealing with.

So these are the basics! Remember, nutrition info is always changing. Stay informed and never self-diagnose. As with any book, our advice is general! You should always check with a physician or dietitian before radically changing your diet.

BIG FAT FAT GLOSSARY

~~~~~~

THE BAD GUYS

Saturated fat increases cholesterol levels and should be eaten minimally. It is found primarily in animal products but does show up in tropical plants such as coconut and palm. Vegan movie theater popcorn is loaded with saturated fat! Most plant-based foods, though, are low in saturated fat.

Trans fats (from hydrogenated oil). This is the chemical processed fat I was talking about. Created by pumping hydrogen into oils to make them shelf stable, these fats mimic saturated fats in their negative health effects. They're found in some margarine, peanut butter, and many commercially packaged baked goods—think all your childhood favorite treats that will never disintegrate, such as Twinkies. Trans fats do not naturally occur in plants, and this book is totally trans-fat free!

~~~~~~

THE GOOD GUYS

Monounsaturated. The heart-healthy fat is found in nuts, avocados, and vegetable oils such as olive and canola. Use in moderation.

Polyunsaturated. Essential nutrients for health; you need these fats the same way you need iron and vitamin D. They're found in soybeans, nuts, seeds—especially flaxseeds—and some leafy green vegetables such as kale. Omega-3 and omega-6 fats are in this category and have additional health benefits.

Omega-3 and omega-6 fatty acids. Omega-3 and omega-6 are types of polyunsaturated fat—the kind you absolutely have to have for growth, reproduction, healthy skin, and more. It's been shown to improve HDL (good cholesterol) and help to lower high blood pressure. It's also especially important for pregnant women or women who are nursing.

When you hear "Omega-3s" you may think of fish, but fish are actually getting their omega-3s from algae, and you can too, in the form of supplements. Algae is not the only source of Omega-3s. Flax seeds and flax oil, walnuts, and kale are all good sources.

About the Recipe Icons

These icons pertain to the individual recipes, not including the serving suggestions.

G Gluten-free: No wheat, or other gluten-containing flours such as rye and barley. We can't vouch for ingredients that might contain gluten on a very small scale, such as oats that aren't labeled gluten free, but the major offenders have been accounted for in these recipes. Several of the recipes marked "can be made gluten free" call for soy sauce, so make sure to use gluten-free tamari as we suggest. And always check your ingredient labels to make sure.

S Soy-free: Recipe doesn't include tofu, tempeh, soy milk, soy sauce, edamame, or any other soy-derived product. Always check labels on items like vegetable broth to make sure.

30 30 minutes or under: For when you need dinner on the table pronto. Of course not everyone cooks at the same pace, but if you know where all your spices are and aren't distracted by crying babies or *Dancing with the Stars*, you should be able to complete these recipes in 30 minutes or less. If you're a little bit slower than that, remember practice makes perfect!

D Downtime: These are some of my favorite weeknight recipes, even more so than the faster recipes; prep is generally easier. Downtime simply means that you have 20 minutes or more where you don't have to do a thing, and dinner is either peacefully simmering away on the stove or baking away in the oven.

One more thing! About cooking spray: I call for non-stick cooking spray in many of the recipes. Of course that "0" calorie info on the label is a big lie. In cases where the spray is absolutely required, I worked an extra teaspoon of oil into the nutritional info. According to one brand's website, there is 1 gram of fat and 7 calories in a one second spray. So if you're using a careful hand and not spraying like a graffiti artist, then don't worry about it.

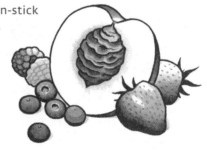

CHAPTER 1

Full-On Salads

THERE WAS A TIME—A LONELY, LONELY TIME—WHEN SALADS were a pale and limp affair, relegated to the side of your plate, practically weeping. I think those dark days were also known as the '80s. Then all of a sudden, salads came alive. Rich dressings, sumptuous vinegars, toasted nuts, roasted veggies, beans, grains, berries . . . the line between salad and entrée was blurred. The walls came down, the arugula came up.

Salads are only as good as their ingredients, so choose the freshest, brightest vegetables you can. That may sound like obvious advice, but just take it as a reminder not to just rush through the produce aisle, grabbing lettuces and tomatoes devil-may-care. Instead, stroll around, touch the produce, smell it, make sure it's the most vivid color it can be. After a while you'll notice that the lettuce bin has become *your* domain and people are asking you questions like, "Is this arugula or spinach?" Roll your eyes and tell them to read the label. Your good deed is done for the day.

But for real, salads can be real meals if you treat them as such. Not "real meals" like how supermodels consider cigarettes and lemon water a real meal, but truly satisfying real meals, the kind that make you lick your plate and dream about leftovers.

The salads in this chapter are mere suggestions for flavors and textures that I think pair well. I've listed the dressings as individual recipes, as a reminder that you can play around and create your own salads out of components in this book, or out of the ingredients you already know and love. And of course you can just pour the dressings over some greens and enjoy (just because salads *can* be entrées doesn't mean they always have to be). Sometimes it's nice to time travel back to those days when haircuts were asymmetrical, Axl ruled the airwaves, and a salad was just a salad.

Anatomy of a Salad (or, the Salad Dissected)

DRESSING UP AND DRESSING DOWN

For many of us, the dressing is our downfall. It's become a cliché that a typical American salad can have more fat and calories than a burger and fries. And sadly, low-fat salad dressings are often chock-full of chemicals and sugar, and boy, does it ever show. I've had upward of ten bottles of low-fat dressing languishing in my refrigerator door, barely used, unwanted, unloved. So I finally gave up even trying and now my dressings are exclusively homemade. Does it take a little extra time? Yes, but usually no more than ten minutes. Is it worth it? Oh, heck yes.

I take a few approaches to salad dressings to get the most out of the ingredients without adding lots of oil. Pureed nuts—especially raw cashews—are my secret weapon in many of the recipes. Nuts have several benefits that oils lack. From a health angle, nuts are a whole food, containing fiber, omega-3s, nutrients, and protein. They also bring big flavor to the dressing, especially if they're toasted first, as in the **Romesco Dressing** (page 47). And to top it all off (literally!) pureeing nuts give dressings excellent texture: smooth and creamy, with plenty of body. Nuts emulsify the dressing naturally, without needing to add any sugars, chemicals, or eggs. The amount of oil you'd need to accomplish all this wouldn't make it one step into a low-fat cookbook before getting bounced out by security.

Speaking of emulsifying, all that means is that you're mixing liquids of varying viscosity, so that they combine without separating. I'm sure you've seen how easily ingredients in dressings separate, but they just need a unifier to bring them together. Nuts are one means, mustard is another, but I often use miso as well. In addition to thickening and emulsifying, miso brings a backdrop of deep, savory flavor to dressings. I like to keep a variety of misos on hand, but I'm kind of an ingredient hoarder. For everyone else, just keep a small tub of a mild white miso that you can use for anything and ignore my specifications for a particular kind. What do I know, anyway?

There is one recipe here that calls for silken tofu. That isn't for everyone—in fact, only recently has it become for me—but when cool and creamy is your calling, a shelf-stable vacuum pack of silken tofu is a pretty handy tool.

I use different vinegars for the dressings, because vinegars are a relatively inexpensive way to bring flavors and nuance to your dressings. Dressings need acidity, but I try not to overdo it. Add small amounts at a time to get a dressing to your "Mmmm" place. Just remember, with vinegars it takes about a second to go from "Mmmm" to "Ewwww." So practice restraint when straying from the recipes and experimenting with vinegars, but definitely do experiment and find a vinegar that you love. I dig white balsamic, but maybe champagne vinegar is your calling? Play around and see.

And as I say throughout the book, this is a low-fat collection, not a no-fat collection. I use such ingredients as peanuts and tahini because not only do they add a world of flavor, but a little fat actually helps you to absorb the nutrients in your food. So, I repeat, don't be fat-phobic with your salads!

But Where Do You Get Your Protein?

Although even greens contain small amounts of protein, it usually takes something more to help us feel full and energized. Many of these salads already contain protein-rich ingredients such as beans, quinoa, nuts, and tofu. But whether you want to make up your own combo or add protein to one of the salads in this chapter, there are lots of great ways to bulk up your bowl.

Whether it's from a can of beans I opened and rinsed, or from dried beans I simmered myself, I always keep handfuls of cooked legumes at the ready in small containers in my fridge. Some of my favorite salad beans are chickpea, kidney, and cannellini—all sturdy beans that hold their shape when they're tossed around. Switch it up and keep things interesting.

I sometimes just cube some tofu and throw it into my salad, but I'm hard-core like that; the rest of the world might not be able to handle it. If you're like the rest of the world, you can try thinly sliced grilled or baked tofu in your salads. Keep leftovers stored in airtight zippered plastic bags; they taste great cold. Same goes for tempeh.

Quinoa is my favorite salad grain. Because it cooks up and cools down so fast, it's as convenient as can be, and I try to keep some cooked quinoa hanging around at all times. I also love the texture of quinoa in salads; it's got a slight chewiness that makes it fun to munch away on, and it also extends the flavors of the dressing, being so small and absorbent. It doesn't hurt that it's a complete protein!

> ∾ TIP *To cool quinoa quickly, place cooked quinoa in a fine mesh strainer and toss it for a minute or so to reduce some of the steam. Place it in the freezer and toss every few minutes. It should be salad-ready in about 15 minutes.* ∾

Nuts give salads great crunch. Because of their high fat and calorie content, I use them in moderation, a few tablespoons at a time. Sliced almonds are a great deal—because they are so thinly sliced, a little goes a long way. They're especially excellent toasted, as in the **Catalan Couscous Salad with Pears** (page 47). I also love cashew pieces, toasted walnuts and pecans, and toasted pine nuts. A sprinkling of sesame seeds goes a long way, too.

A Berry for Your Thoughts

Fruit is a great addition to salads, especially with very vinegary dressings. The acid brings out the sweetness of the fruit in unexpected ways. I admit to not getting incredibly adventurous with fruits in salad—the usual suspects do a pretty good job, especially when they're in season. You won't see me putting cantaloupe or bananas in my salad—but hey, maybe you'd love that! My favorite fruits to use are sliced strawberries, whole raspberries and blackberries, sliced pears and apples, and orange segments (learn how to get pretty orange segments in the **Wild Rice Salad with Oranges & Roasted Beets**, page 39). When the season is right, make a day of it and go berry picking or have a blast at an apple orchard. You haven't lived until you've tasted a strawberry fresh-plucked and still warm from the morning sun. You'll also get in some exercise and save a couple of bucks. Win win win!

Lettuce Begin

When we come to greens, this is really where you can see how much the supermarket has changed in the past twenty years or so. Crotchety old man voice: "In my day, we had a head of plastic-wrapped iceberg lettuce and a bag of coleslaw mix and we liked it!" But when it comes to the produce aisle, even Kansas ain't in Kansas anymore.

I do call for a variety of salad greens in this chapter, but instead of taking you step by step through every curvy, frilly, silky, crispy, and otherwise sexy variety of lettuce, I'll just tell you this—try them all at least once! Salad greens have as much nuance as wine and supermarkets vary year-round in what kinds they keep in stock. Taste the greens and detect the different notes: bitter, spicy, sweet, mellow. There are worlds of flavor in that leaf.

That said, my go-to everyday lettuce is romaine, with a little arugula thrown in when I want to spice things up. Sure, it's not all that exciting, but I enjoy the crispiness and convenience of it.

The Usual Suspects

I love seedless cucumbers, orange grape tomatoes when they're in season, all manner of sprouts, especially broccoli and alfalfa, sliced cremini mushrooms, and when it comes to onions, make mine red: you just can't beat their crisp, sweet bite. New and fun radishes are popping up at farmers' markets and it never hurts to add a few for a little spice and color.

> ∾ TIP *If you've got some yard space or even just a big container with some drainage holes, it might be a good idea to plant some lettuce in the spring-time. It's such a delicious and economical choice, because you can pull the leaves off as you need them, without killing the plant. They'll keep growing back and keeping you happy throughout summer. Forget "farm to table"; how about porch to table?* ∾

Tools of the Trade

As far as equipment goes, I'm willing to make a few more dirty dishes if it means it will make my salad all that much more lip-smacking.

A **huge metal mixing bowl** is my vessel of choice, for tossing together ingredients and getting everything evenly coated. Use a pair of metal tongs, and toss like the pros!

Because you're making relatively small batches of dressings at a time, a **small food processor** is necessary to blend the party up nice and creamy. I'm pretty sold on the Magic Bullet. Full disclosure: A tester for this book turned me on to it and now I find it indispensible. The reason I love it so is not just that it gets the job done quickly, cleanly, and efficiently, but it comes with several containers that can be used not only for blending, but also you can store the dressings right in them; no need to transfer to Tupperware. Several lids and containers with handles (meant, I think, to make margaritas in) make it possible to store a variety of dressings all at once. It's a small kind of very convenient heaven, as seen on TV.

Not completely necessary, a **salad spinner** is great to keep washed lettuces crisp and dry and ready for any dressing you choose to throw at it. It also doubles as a colander! Consider picking one up when you're ready to make salads with deadly precision.

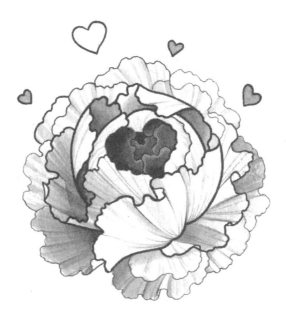

Everyday Chickpea-Quinoa Salad

SERVES 4 • ACTIVE TIME: 10 MINUTES • TOTAL TIME: 10 MINUTES
IF QUINOA IS PREPPED, IF NOT THEN 1 HOUR

PER SERVING
(¼ RECIPE):
Calories: 290
Calories from fat: 55
Total fat: 6 g
Saturated fat: 1 g
Trans fat: 0 g
Total carb: 49 g
Fiber: 11 g
Sugars: 6 g
Protein: 12 g
Cholesterol: 0 mg
Sodium: 618 mg
Vitamin A: 85%
Vitamin C: 23%
Calcium: 8%
Iron: 20%

I call this Everyday Chickpea-Quinoa Salad for a very simple reason: I eat it almost every day! Not only is it a complete meal, it's everything I want in a salad—texture, nutrients, and ease, all smothered in an irresistible balsamic vinaigrette. It's also foreverly customizable: switch up your salad greens, your beans, and even the grain. Try it my way once, then use this as your complete meal salad template.

This salad makes use of cooked and cooled quinoa, so make your quinoa the day before and you're good to go. Otherwise, use the grain cooking and cooling tips on pages 13 and 76.

2 cups cooked, cooled quinoa (pages 13, 76)
1 small red onion, sliced thinly
4 cups chopped romaine lettuce
1 (15-ounce) can chickpeas, drained and rinsed
   Optional add-ins: roasted garlic, baked tofu or tempeh, shredded carrot, sprouts, fresh basil
1 recipe **Balsamic Vinaigrette** (recipe follows)

In a large mixing bowl, mix all the salad ingredients together. Add the dressing and toss to coat. Keep chilled in a tightly sealed container for up to 3 days.

Balsamic Vinaigrette

SERVES 4; MAKES ¾ CUP DRESSING • ACTIVE TIME: 10 MINUTES • TOTAL TIME: 10 MINUTES

Don't roll your eyes at balsamic vinaigrette. There's a reason this dressing is everywhere—it's addictively delicious. There is always a little container of this in my fridge, and if you're wise you will follow my lead! As with all cashew-based dressings, if you've got the time, soak the cashews in water for at least an hour. Then drain them and use as directed. This makes blending easier and smoother.

> ¼ cup cashew pieces (see tip page 38)
> 2 tablespoons chopped shallot
> ½ cup water
> ¼ cup balsamic vinegar
> 2 teaspoons Dijon mustard
> 1 teaspoon agave nectar
> ¾ teaspoon salt
> A few pinches of freshly ground black pepper

PER SERVING (ABOUT 3 TABLESPOONS):
Calories: 75
Calories from fat: 35
Total fat: 4 g
Saturated fat: 1 g
Trans fat: 0 g
Total carb: 8 g
Fiber: 0 g
Sugars: 4 g
Protein: 2 g
Cholesterol: 0 mg
Sodium: 502 mg
Vitamin A: 1%
Vitamin C: 1%
Calcium: 1%
Iron: 4%

First place the cashews and shallot in a food processor and pulse to get them chopped up. Then simply add the rest of the ingredients. Blend for at least 5 minutes, using a rubber spatula to scrape down the sides often, until completely smooth. It's really important that you blend for the full time, otherwise your dressing may be grainy. Transfer the dressing to a sealable container (a bowl covered with plastic wrap is just fine!) and chill until ready to serve.

> ∾ NOTE *This dressing may seem thin at first, but it thickens as it chills.* ∾

Spicy Blue Potato & Corn Salad

SERVES 6 • ACTIVE TIME: 20 MINUTES • TOTAL TIME: 45 MINUTES, PLUS COOLING TIME

~~~~~~~~~~~~~~~~~~
PER SERVING
(⅙ RECIPE):
Calories: 280
Calories from fat: 25
Total fat: 3 g
Saturated fat: 0 g
Trans fat: 0 g
Fiber: 11 g
Protein: 12 g
Cholesterol: 0 mg
Sodium: 115 mg
Vitamin A: 4%
Vitamin C: 60%
Calcium: 6%
Iron: 20%

This salad is so deliciously complex with its fun textures, colors, and smoky spicy flavor that you won't miss that goopy potato salad present at every family function. And with fresh corn and pinto beans, it's so much healthier, too. If you can't find blue potatoes, just use red! The firmer texture works better with this salad, and you want to keep things colorful. This recipe also contains a hidden treasure, the secret to perfectly cooked, salad-ready potatoes. The answer is "steaming."

3 ears corn, shucked
2 pounds blue potatoes, peeled and cut into ½-inch pieces
3 tablespoons red wine vinegar
2 canned chipotles, seeded and mashed into a paste (see tips)
2 tablespoons adobo sauce from chipotle can (see tips)
2 teaspoons grapeseed oil
1 teaspoon light agave nectar
2 tablespoons water
¼ teaspoon salt
1 teaspoon garlic, grated on a Microplane grater or minced very well
1 (16-ounce) can pinto beans, drained and rinsed
2 tablespoons finely chopped red onion
¼ cup chopped fresh cilantro
Mixed greens, for serving
Smoked paprika (optional)

Prepare your steaming apparatus while you prep your veggies.

First, steam the corn for about 5 minutes. Remove from the steamer and set aside until cool enough to handle.

Place the potatoes in the steamer, and steam for 7 to 10 minutes. The potatoes should be tender enough to pierce with a fork, but not falling apart. Remove from the steamer and set aside to cool.

In the meantime, prepare the dressing. In a small mixing bowl, stir together vinegar, chipotles, adobo, oil, agave, water, and salt. Grate in the garlic.

When the corn is cool enough to handle, cut it from the cob: Place it directly in a large mixing bowl, pointy side up, and use your chef's knife to cut down the sides. Once all the corn is in there, just break it up with your fingers. Fold in the cooled potatoes, pinto beans, and red onion.

> ∾ TIP Bored with fresh, healthy food? Well, add a little excitement by burning your tongue off! I kid, but spicy food really does make you forget that what you're eating is low fat. ℯ∾

Add the dressing and toss to coat. Mix in the cilantro and taste for salt. Chipotles in adobe vary from brand to brand, so if it doesn't seem smoky enough for you, rather than add more chipotle and risk overheating, add some smoked paprika and see if that doesn't fix it to your liking. Start with a teaspoon and go from there. Chill until ready to serve. Serve over the mixed greens.

> ∾ TIP If you avoid the seeds in the can of chipotles, then this salad is only mildly spicy. To remove seeds from chipotles, split them in half and use a paring knife to scrape the seeds out. When spooning up the adobo sauce, avoid the seeds or pick them out with tweezers. To mash your chipotle, you can use a mortar and pestle, but since you don't want to dust that old thing off, you can also just chop it with your chef's knife and then mash it with the side of the blade. ℯ∾

Sushi Roll Edamame Salad

SERVES 4 • ACTIVE TIME: 15 MINUTES • TOTAL TIME: 20 MINUTES

PER SERVING
(¼ RECIPE):
Calories: 280
Calories from fat: 60
Total fat: 7 g
Saturated fat: 1 g
Trans fat: 0 g
Total carb: 47 g
Fiber: 10 g
Sugars: 8 g
Protein: 9 g
Cholesterol: 0 mg
Sodium: 670 mg
Vitamin A: 230%
Vitamin C: 70%
Calcium: 20%
Iron: 25%
1 serving of optional
avocado (1 ounce) adds
45 calories, 4 grams
of fat (mostly mono-
unsaturated), and 2
grams of fiber.

Eating this salad is a good time. How many salads can you say that about? It's just fun! As the name indicates, it's basically a big, deconstructed sushi roll in a bowl. Make a point to have leftover brown rice in the fridge and this will come together in a snap. If you like, serve this with a lump of wasabi and soy sauce on the side and dip in each bite, using chopsticks, of course. The cooking times include prepping the dressing, which you should actually do first, before beginning the rest of the salad.

- 1 cup shelled frozen edamame, thawed
- 1 tablespoon rice vinegar
- 1 teaspoon light agave nectar
- 8 cups chopped romaine lettuce
- 2 cups cooked and cooled short-grain brown rice
- 1 small cucumber, cut into matchsticks
- 1 medium-size carrot, cut into matchsticks
- 1 cup thinly sliced green onion
- 4 teaspoons sesame seeds
- 1 sheet nori, chiffonaded
- 4 ounces sliced avocado (optional)
- 1 recipe **Green Onion–Miso Vinaigrette** (recipe follows)

Prepare the dressing: Mix together the edamame, rice vinegar, and agave. Now you're ready to assemble the salad.

Place the lettuce in a bowl and drizzle with a little dressing. Scoop the rice over the lettuce. Top the rice with the cucumber, carrot, green onion, and sesame seeds. Sprinkle with the nori chiffonade and avocado, if using, and serve with the vinaigrette on the side.

> **TIP** Chiffonade *just means "cut into superthin strips." To achieve this, roll up the nori sheet into a cylinder and then thinly slice. You'll get pretty little ribbons of nori that look great on top of salad.*

Green Onion–Miso Vinaigrette

SERVES 4 • ACTIVE TIME: 10 MINUTES • TOTAL TIME: 10 MINUTES

I want to cover everything with this brilliant spring green dressing. Roasted veggies, steamed potatoes, my cat . . . everything. Green onions and scallions are often confused for each other or labeled interchangeably but they're actually *not* the same exact thing. If you can find green onions (sometimes called spring onions) then use them! You can tell them apart because green onions have a bulbuous white bottom (don't you love the phrase "bulbous white bottom"?) from which the green stalks grow. Scallions, on the other hand, have no bulb, just roots, and the stalks are hollow. I prefer the snappy taste of green onion here, but scallions will do just fine, too!

¼	cup red miso
1 to 2	cups roughly chopped green onions, white and green parts
3	tablespoons rice vinegar
2	teaspoons chopped fresh ginger
1	clove garlic
2	teaspoons light agave nectar
2	teaspoons toasted sesame oil
½ to ¾	cup water

This is easy: Toss everything into a blender and blend until smooth. At first, use just ½ cup of water, adding the ¼ cup after the dressing is blended, to desired thinness. Use a rubber spatula to scrape down the sides occasionally. Chill until ready to use.

PER SERVING
(ABOUT ¼ CUP):
Calories: 80
Calories from fat: 20
Total fat: 2.5 g
Saturated fat: 0 g
Trans fat: 0 g
Total carb: 11 g
Fiber: 3 g
Sugars: 3 g
Protein: <1 g
Cholesterol: 0 mg
Sodium: 640 mg
Vitamin A: 10%
Vitamin C: 15%
Calcium: 6%
Iron: 4%

> **NOTE** *The recipe calls for 1 to 2 cups of chopped green onion because the strength of your onions can vary so much. So start with the cup and after your initial blending, see if it could use a bit more.*

Big Fat Taco Salad

SERVES 4 • ACTIVE TIME: 20 MINUTES • TOTAL TIME: 20 MINUTES

PER SERVING
(¼ RECIPE):
Calories: 350
Calories from fat: 60
Total fat: 6 g
Saturated fat: 1 g
Trans fat: 0 g
Total carb: 59 g
Fiber: 16 g
Sugars: 6 g
Protein: 17 g
Cholesterol: 0 mg
Sodium: 300 mg
Vitamin A: 110%
Vitamin C: 60%
Calcium: 10%
Iron: 25%

There are lots of variations on taco salad, but one thing is certain—it's got to be big and fat. This version uses low-fat baked corn tortilla chips for crunch, black beans for the meaty component, shredded lettuce (obviously), a fresh tomato salsa dressing for big taco flavors, and what taco salad would be complete without guacamole? Here, we use my slimmed-down version called Guacamame. To make the tortilla chips go a long way, I crumble them a bit over the top, kinda like croutons. If your taco salad is not complete without something cool and creamy, you can also use a bit of **Sanctuary Dressing** (page 29), if you like.

    4 cups shredded romaine lettuce
    1 (15-ounce) can black beans, drained and rinsed
    1 recipe **Fresh Tomato Salsa Dressing** (recipe follows)
    4 ounces low-fat baked tortilla chips
    ½ cup chopped fresh cilantro
    4 servings **Guacamame** (about 1 cup, recipe follows)

Arrange the salad among four big bowls: First place the lettuce in the bowls, then layer on the beans and salsa. Crumble on the tortilla chips and top with the cilantro. Serve with Guacamame on the side.

Fresh Tomato Salsa Dressing

SERVES 4 • ACTIVE TIME: 5 MINUTES • TOTAL TIME: 5 MINUTES

This is called salsa *dressing*, so it isn't exactly salsa, more of a piquant and zesty dressing, perfect for salad greens and beans alike. Bonus: it's completely fat free!

- 1 pound tomatoes (about 3 average-size guys)
- ¼ cup chopped fresh cilantro
- 1 clove garlic, minced
- 1 tablespoon red wine vinegar
- 2 teaspoons cayenne hot sauce
  Freshly ground black pepper
- ⅛ teaspoon salt, or to taste

Chop up the tomatoes fairly small, placing them immediately in a mixing bowl so that not much liquid escapes. Add the remaining ingredients and use your hands to mush everything up really well. Let sit for 10 minutes or so to let the flavors meld. Chill in a tightly sealed container until ready to use, for up to 5 days.

PER SERVING
(ABOUT ½ CUP):
Calories: 25
Calories from fat: 0
Total fat: 0 g
Saturated fat: 0 g
Trans fat: 0 g
Total carb: 5 g
Fiber: 1 g
Sugars: 3 g
Protein: 1 g
Cholesterol: 0 mg
Sodium: 80 mg
Vitamin A: 25%
Vitamin C: 25%
Calcium: 0%
Iron: 2%

Guacamame

SERVES 6; MAKES 1½ CUPS • ACTIVE TIME: 15 MINUTES • TOTAL TIME: 15 MINUTES

There are lots of recipes online for mock guacamole made out of asparagus or artichokes, and I've tried those, but really all they do is make me crave guacamole. I prefer guac the way God intended—with avocados! This version uses a mixture of avocado with edamame to cut the fat a bit but still give you that succulent, sexy avo goodness that you crave. It's not quite as smooth as pure avocado guac, but it gets the job done. Make sure to thaw your edamame for 12 hours before making this recipe, or thaw it in the microwave or by running under warm water.

4 ounces sliced avocado
1 cup frozen edamame, completely thawed
¼ cup water
¼ teaspoon salt
Juice of 1 lime
1 plum tomato, chopped
2 tablespoons chopped red onion
¼ cup loosely packed cilantro leaves (optional)
Pinch of cayenne, for spiciness (optional)

Place the avocado and edamame in a food processor. Pulse until everything is well chopped. Add the water, salt, and lime juice, and puree until relatively smooth, scraping down the sides with a spatula to make sure you get everything. Add the tomato, red onion, cilantro, and cayenne, if using, and pulse a bit, just to get the onion and tomatoes finely chopped and incorporated. Remove from the food processor, and taste for salt and seasoning. Serve ASAP.

∾ TIP *To keep Guacamame from turning brown, throw the avocado pit into the 'mame, drizzle with extra lime juice, and lay a piece of plastic wrap right on the surface of the mixture. Then, cover tightly with plastic wrap and refrigerate.* ∾

Goddess Niçoise

SERVES 4 • ACTIVE TIME: 20 MINUTES • TOTAL TIME: 30 MINUTES

Salade Niçoise is a bistro staple. It's steamed potatoes, crisp green beans, and salty Niçoise olives dunked in a lush dressing. Traditionally it is served with tuna, but I serve it with lightly mashed chickpeas that are spiked with briny capers. NYC sidewalk cafés are lined with ladies talking on their cell phones, reading French *Vogue*, and eating this salad. Now you can bring it home, *sans* all the bus exhaust in your face and the crazy drunk guy trying to steal the bread basket off your table.

Green Goddess Garlic Dressing is a perfect accompaniment, but you can also serve it with the more traditional **Balsamic Vinaigrette** (page 17) if you prefer. Tiny red potatoes work best here, but if you can't find any, then chop up regular ones into 1-inch pieces. This recipe does make a bunch of dirty dishes, but be a goddess and have someone else clean them up! For time-management purposes, prepare the dressing while the potatoes are steaming, or (even better) prepare the dressing a day in advance.

PER SERVING
(¼ RECIPE):
Calories: 250
Calories from fat: 60
Total fat: 7 g
Saturated fat: 0 g
Trans fat: 0 g
Total carb: 38 g
Fiber: 10 g
Sugars: 6 g
Protein: 11 g
Cholesterol: 0 mg
Sodium: 810 mg
Vitamin A: 110%
Vitamin C: 60%
Calcium: 10%
Iron: 25%

    1 (16-ounce) can chickpeas, drained and rinsed
    2 tablespoons capers
    ½ pound small whole red potatoes
    ½ pound green beans, stems removed
    ½ small red onion, cut into thin strips
    ⅓ cup Niçoise olives (kalamata olives work, too)
    8 cups chopped red leaf lettuce
    1 cup cherry tomatoes (orange ones if you can get them)
       Fresh parsley and chopped chives, for garnish
       About ¾ cup **Green Goddess Garlic Dressing** (recipe follows)

Prepare your steamer for the potatoes. Once it's ready, steam the potatoes for 10 to 15 minutes; they should be pierced easily with a fork. Meanwhile, prepare an ice bath by filling a mixing bowl halfway with ice water. Add the green beans to the steamer and steam for 2 more minutes, until the beans are bright green.

Transfer the potatoes and green beans to the ice bath immediately. Let them cool while you prepare everything else.

Place the chickpeas in a mixing bowl and use a small potato masher or a fork to mash them. There should be no whole chickpeas left, but they shouldn't be completely smooth like hummus, either; you want some texture. Add the capers and 2 tablespoons of the dressing. Mix well and set aside.

To assemble, place the lettuce in wide bowls. In a Salade Niçoise, usually all the components are kept together, instead of tossed. Place a handful each of potatoes and green beans in piles on the lettuce, along with a wedge of sliced onion and a handful of tomatoes. Place a scoop of the chickpea mixture in the center and top with the olives. Garnish with fresh herbs and serve with the dressing on the side.

Green Goddess Garlic Dressing

SERVES 6 (3 TABLESPOONS EACH) • ACTIVE TIME: 15 MINUTES • TOTAL TIME: 15 MINUTES

PER SERVING
(ABOUT 3
TABLESPOONS):
Calories: 45
Calories from fat: 25
Total fat: 3 g
Saturated fat: 0 g
Trans fat: 0 g
Total carb: 4 g
Fiber: 1 g
Sugars: 0 g
Protein: 2 g
Cholesterol: 0 mg
Sodium: 320 mg
Vitamin A: 10%
Vitamin C: 20%
Calcium: 2%
Iron: 4%

This is the stuff! I don't use the word mouthwatering lightly, but the moment this dressing touches my tongue it just permeates every taste bud, and perhaps even the very core of my being. Herby, garlicky, tangy, luscious, vibrant . . . I'm gonna burn out all my food adjectives if I go on. I love to pour it on grain and bean salads. The tahini makes it a natural player in a Middle Eastern spread, and the miso makes it equally at home with Japanese dishes. But really, with all the flavors going on, it's kind of everyone's best friend. Again, use whichever miso you have on hand.

2 to 3 average-size cloves garlic
½ cup fresh chives
½ cup fresh parsley
2 tablespoons tahini
2 tablespoons nutritional yeast
1 tablespoon miso

⅓ cup water

2 tablespoons freshly squeezed lemon juice

½ teaspoon salt

Pulse two cloves of garlic, the chives, and the parsley in a food processor just to chop everything up. Add the remaining ingredients and blend until very smooth. Use a rubber spatula to scrape down the sides a few times. Now you should adjust it to your liking. See if it needs more salt and garlic, and thin the dressing with a tablespoon or two of water, if needed. Note that it will thicken a bit as it's refrigerated, so if it appears thin, don't worry!

Transfer to a tightly sealed container and chill until ready to serve.

ᰍ NOTE

This salad doesn't call for the entire recipe of the goddess dressing; reserve the rest for sandwiches the next day. ᰍ

Sanctuary Chef Salad

SERVES 4 • ACTIVE TIME: 30 MINUTES • TOTAL TIME: 1 HOUR (TO ALLOW THINGS TO COOL DOWN)

~~~~~~~~~~~~~~
PER SERVING
(¼ CUP):
Calories: 190
Calories from fat: 60
Total fat: 7 g
Saturated fat: 1 g
Trans fat: 0 g
Total carb: 25 g
Fiber: 9 g
Sugars: 12 g
Protein: 12 g
Cholesterol: 0 mg
Sodium: 930 mg
Vitamin A: 230%
Vitamin C: 140%
Calcium: 20%
Iron: 20%

This is the kind of salad that deserves to be eaten in the biggest bowl you've got. Lots of pretty veggies are just bursting with color, and this contains all the chef's favorite meats: eggplant bacon, baked tofu, and roasted cauliflower. Don't expect to be hungry for a few hours after eating this big boy. Make some components in advance, bake the tofu and roast the cauliflower at the same time, and it's smooth sailing (or, cheffing) from there. If you can't find sunflower sprouts, broccoli sprouts or alfalfa sprouts will work, too.

  8 cups chopped romaine lettuce
  ½ recipe **Herb-Roasted Cauliflower,** cooled (page 108)
  1 recipe **Eggplant Bacon** (page 42)
  ½ recipe **Basic Baked Tofu,** cooled, cut into bite-size pieces (page 144)
  1 cup thinly sliced radishes
  1 small red onion, sliced thinly
  1 cup sunflower sprouts
1½ cups cherry tomatoes
  1 medium-size carrot, peeled and shredded
  ½ recipe **Sanctuary Dressing** (recipe follows)

Basically, just toss everything together, or arrange however you prefer.

Sanctuary Dressing

SERVES 8 • ACTIVE TIME: 10 MINUTES • TOTAL TIME: 10 MINUTES

Because ranches are not nice places for cows, I give you Sanctuary Dressing. I fussed with this recipe a lot, trying to achieve something rich and creamy, the stuff you wanna just drink from the bottle, without having a gazillion grams of fat. The litmus test is, "Do I lick it off the spatula and am I reluctant to put the food processor in the sink until I have gotten every last bit?" A resolute yes!

PER SERVING
(SCANT ¼ CUP):
Calories: 40
Calories from fat: 25
Total fat: 2.5 g
Saturated fat: 0 g
Trans fat: 0 g
Total carb: 2 g
Fiber: 0 g
Sugars: <1 g
Protein: 2 g
Cholesterol: 0 mg
Sodium: 130 mg
Vitamin A: 0%
Vitamin C: 0%
Calcium: 4%
Iron: 2%

- 12 ounces extra-firm silken tofu (the vacuum-packed kind, such as Mori-Nu), cut into 1-inch cubes
- 2 tablespoons reduced-fat vegan mayonaisse
- ¼ cup water
- 2 tablespoons vegetable broth powder
- ¼ teaspoon salt
- 1 teaspoon garlic powder
- 1 teaspoon onion flakes
- 2 tablespoons apple cider vinegar
- 1 teaspoon light agave nectar
  Pinch of freshly ground black pepper
- ¼ cup lightly packed fresh dill, or 1 teaspoon dried

First we're going to blanch the tofu, but don't be deterred by a little stove-top action. It will take only a few minutes and you can gather everything else while the water is coming to a boil. This step is important because it takes away the "beany" taste associated with blended tofu.

Bring a small pot of water to a boil, just enough to submerge the tofu in. When boiling, add the tofu and cover. Lower the heat to a simmer and

> **NOTE** *This dressing is thick, and it thickens even more as it chills. If you prefer a thinner dressing, just dilute with tablespoonfuls of unsweetened nondairy milk. You may have to adjust the seasonings a bit so that the flavor is not diluted, but that shouldn't be a big deal.*

let cook for 2 minutes. Drain into a colander and run under cold water for 30 seconds or so, just to cool it down a bit.

In a food processor or blender, combine the tofu, mayo, and water. Blend until smooth, scraping down the sides with a rubber spatula to make sure you get everything.

Add the remaining ingredients, except for the dill if you're using fresh, and blend until smooth. Taste for salt. Add the fresh dill and pulse until it's just tiny flecks of green in the dressing.

Transfer the dressing to a container, cover tightly, and chill until ready to use. It tastes even better after it's chilled a few hours. Keeps well for about 3 days.

೦ INGREDIENT SCAVENGER HUNT

A few words about the ingredients: If reduced-fat Vegenaise is not available to you, you can use full-fat vegan mayo; just try 1 tablespoon plus 1 teaspoon at first and see if that does the trick for you. It's diluted enough in this dressing that even if you need 2 tablespoons, it should still fit into your food budget. I even tried it with 1 tablespoon of grapeseed oil instead, and it was good, but the Vegenaise makes it great. As for the broth powder, it really does great things for the texture so I decided to use it. Some brands I like are Vogue VegeBase and Frontier veg broth or nonchicken broth powder. ೦

Quinoa Salad with Black Beans & Toasted Cumin Seeds

SERVES 4 • ACTIVE TIME: 15 MINUTES • TOTAL TIME: 15 MINUTES IF QUINOA IS PREPPED, OTHERWISE 45 MINUTES

I can't get enough of quinoa salad during the summer. As I keep mentioning, when you have cooked quinoa in the fridge to use as your heart desires, that makes throwing together salads like this a snap. The toasted cumin seeds bring a delicate smokiness to the salad, and the flavor seeps into the tomatoes and flavors everything. As with most grain salads, the longer you let it sit, the more the flavor will develop, making this salad an "even better the next day" kind of thing. Use red quinoa for the prettiest results.

- 2 cups cooked quinoa (page 76)
- ¼ teaspoon salt
- 2 teaspoons cumin seeds
- 1 cup finely diced plum tomatoes (about 4)
- 3 tablespoons freshly squeezed lime juice (3 to 4 limes)
- 2 teaspoons light agave nectar
- 1 teaspoon grapeseed oil
- 1 (15-ounce) can black beans, drained and rinsed
- 1 cup finely chopped scallions
  Mixed greens, for serving

PER SERVING
(¼ RECIPE):
Calories: 230
Calories from fat: 30
Total fat: 3 g
Saturated fat: 0 g
Trans fat: 0 g
Fiber: 11 g
Protein: 12 g
Cholesterol: 0 mg
Sodium: 110 mg
Vitamin A: 15%
Vitamin C: 30%
Calcium: 10%
Iron: 20%

∿ TIPS

• For a fun presentation, pack a teacup with salad. Gently turn over the cup onto the plate and lift to unmold. Marvel at the fanciness.

• Toasting cumin seeds is a wonderful way to bring out their deep, smoky flavor. Once you try this method you might fall in love and find yourself adding toasted cumin seeds to soups, chilis, and everything but your morning coffee. ∿

Place the quinoa in a large mixing bowl, if it isn't already cooling in one.

To toast the cumin seeds, preheat an 8-inch pan over low heat. Place the cumin seeds in the dry pan and toss often for about 5 minutes. Immediately transfer to a medium-size mixing bowl.

Add the tomatoes, lime juice, agave, and grapeseed oil to the mixing bowl and mix well. When the quinoa has cooled, mix it in. Fold in the beans and scallions. Taste for salt. You can serve immediately or let sit for a bit for the flavors to meld. Serve over the greens.

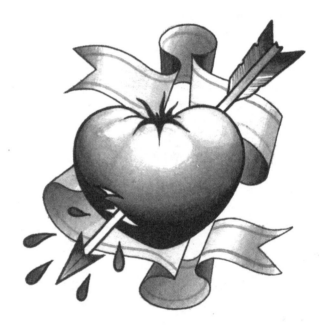

Pad Thai Salad

SERVES 4 • ACTIVE TIME: 15 MINUTES • TOTAL TIME: 15 MINUTES

(CAN BE MADE GLUTEN FREE IF USING GF TAMARI IN PLACE OF SOY SAUCE)

You could eat Pad Thai for dinner every night of the week, and it would be delicious but way too greasy! This salad borrows all of the Pad Thai flavors—sweet, sour, hot and salty—and gives you something to satisfy the Pad Thai urge that you actually *could* eat every night of the week. If you'd like to bulk it up, **Red Thai Tofu** (page 149) makes a natural choice.

- 8 cups chopped romaine lettuce
- 4 cups bean sprouts
- 1 small red onion, sliced thinly
- 1 medium-size carrot, peeled and grated
- 1 recipe **Peanut–Lime Dragon Dressing** (recipe follows)
- ¼ cup roasted peanuts
- ½ cup lightly packed fresh cilantro (stem and leaves)
  Lime wedges, for serving

In a large mixing bowl, toss together the lettuce, sprouts, red onion, and carrot. Add the dressing and toss to coat. Distribute the salad among four bowls. There will be dressing left over because it is fairly thin; distribute the remaining dressing among the bowls. Garnish with the roasted peanuts and cilantro, and serve with the lime wedges.

PER SERVING
(¼ RECIPE):
Calories: 210
Calories from fat: 90
Total fat: 9.5 g
Saturated fat: 1.5 g
Trans fat: 0 g
Total carb: 26 g
Fiber: 7 g
Sugars: 12 g
Protein: 10 g
Cholesterol: 0 mg
Sodium: 570 mg
Vitamin A: 220%
Vitamin C: 80%
Calcium: 15%
Iron: 15%

> ∿ NUTRITION TIP *This salad has peanuts and peanuts have fat. But as mentioned elsewhere in the book, do allow some fat into your plan. Fats help you feel full and satisfied. The protein and fiber of the nuts and bean sprouts help, too. At only 210 calories per serving, the nutrient-to-calorie ratio of this salad is still fantastic, especially considering that most cold peanut salads contain about five times the fat and calories of this one. You don't want to live a life without peanuts! (Unless you're allergic, of course, but if you are, you probably aren't reading this.)* ∿

Peanut–Lime Dragon Dressing

SERVES 4 • ACTIVE TIME: 5 MINUTES • TOTAL TIME: 5 MINUTES

(CAN BE MADE GLUTEN FREE IF USING GF TAMARI IN PLACE OF SOY SAUCE)

Peanut and lime loooove each other, and who am I to keep them apart? Sriracha brings the heat and ties the flavors together and turns you into a fire-breathing dragon! Half the peanuts are blended into the dressing, and the other half of them are left choppy. This extends the peanutty flavor and adds some texture, without having to add a bunch more fat and calories.

- ¼ cup roasted peanuts
- 2 tablespoons chopped shallot
- ¼ cup freshly squeezed lime juice
- ½ cup water
- 2 tablespoons agave nectar
- 2 tablespoons soy sauce
- 1 teaspoon Sriracha, or more if you like it hot

Pulse 2 tablespoons of the peanuts and all of the shallot in the food processor, just to chop everything up. Add the lime juice, water, agave, soy sauce, and Sriracha, and blend until very smooth. Use a rubber spatula to scrape down the sides a few times. Now add the remaining 2 tablespoons of peanuts and pulse for a bit. These shouldn't be blended smooth, just chopped up small. The dressing will be fairly thin. Adjust the seasonings to your liking. Keep refrigerated in a tightly sealed container until ready to use, up to 5 days.

Warm Mushroom Salad with Cranberries

SERVES 4 • ACTIVE TIME: 20 MINUTES • TOTAL TIME: 20 MINUTES

Inspired by one of my favorite restaurants, New York City's Candle Café, this recipe will really give you that accomplished gourmet feeling with hardly any work at all. Earthy mushrooms are gently sautéed, then placed atop delicately flavored mâche greens, tossed in a creamy horseradish dressing, and studded with sweet, dried cranberries. Simple ingredients that deliver flavors that can only be described as *exquisite*, if you're the type to use the word *exquisite*. This would be an excellent Thanksgiving salad and doesn't taste at all low fat, so don't be afraid to serve it to a crowd. It would also be great to serve on a soup-and-salad kind of night.

1 teaspoon olive oil
2 cloves garlic, minced
½ pound chanterelle mushrooms, sliced ¼ inch thick (see note)
¼ teaspoon salt
¼ teaspoon dried thyme
  Freshly ground black pepper
16 ounces mâche greens
½ cup dried sweetened cranberries
1 recipe **Creamy Horseradish Dressing** (recipe follows)

PER SERVING
(¼ RECIPE):
Calories: 150
Calories from fat: 45
Total fat: 5 g
Saturated fat: 0.5 g
Trans fat: 0 g
Total carb: 25 g
Fiber: 2 g
Sugars: 12 g
Protein: 5 g
Cholesterol: 0 mg
Sodium: 350 mg
Vitamin A: 160%
Vitamin C: 80%
Calcium: 6%
Iron: 20%

⟋ INGREDIENT SCAVENGER HUNT

Mâche greens can be hard to find if your supermarket doesn't happen to have a well-stocked gourmet-type yuppie produce aisle. Mâche is also known as "lamb's lettuce." I've never actually seen it labeled that, but it's worth mentioning because it's so cute. If you can't find it, a combination of arugula and green leaf lettuces tastes fantastic, too. Also, just so you don't embarrass yourself in the produce aisle, it's pronounced "mash." ⟋

Preheat a large pan over medium heat. Sauté the garlic in oil for about 30 seconds, then add the mushrooms, salt, pepper, thyme, and a splash of water. Cover the pan to make some of the moisture release from the mushrooms, about 3 minutes. Remove the cover and sauté for about 5 more minutes, flipping often, until the mushrooms are tender.

Remove from the heat.

In a large mixing bowl, toss together the greens and cranberries. Drizzle in the dressing and use tongs to coat thoroughly. Divide among four plates and top with the warm mushrooms. Serve immediately.

> ∾ **TIP** *Prepare the dressing first, and don't bother washing the pan after sautéing for that recipe. Instead, immediate begin sautéeing the mushrooms for the salad.* ∾

Creamy Horseradish Dressing

SERVES 4 • ACTIVE TIME: 15 MINUTES • TOTAL TIME: 15 MINUTES

PER SERVING
(2 TABLESPOONS):
Calories: 50
Calories from fat: 30
Total fat: 3 g
Saturated fat: 0.5 g
Trans fat: 0 g
Total carb: 5 g
Fiber: 0 g
Sugars: 2 g
Protein: 1 g
Cholesterol: 0 mg
Sodium: 190 mg
Vitamin A: 2%
Vitamin C: 4%
Calcium: 0%
Iron: 2%

I'm always looking for ways to use a jar of horseradish, and I'm always looking for ways to punch up the flavor in my dressings. What a convenient coincidence! Sautéeing the shallots for this dressing adds to the creaminess that the cashews bring.

- 1 teaspoon olive oil
- ¼ cup shallot, chopped finely
- 1 clove garlic, minced
- 2 tablespoons raw cashew pieces (see tip about soaked cashews, page 38)
- 4 teaspoons prepared horseradish
- 2 tablespoons water
- 1 teaspoon Dijon mustard
  Freshly ground black pepper
- ¼ teaspoon salt
- 1 tablespoon white balsamic vinegar (sub regular balsamic if you need to)

Preheat a small pan over medium heat. Sauté the shallot and garlic in the oil for about 3 minutes, until the shallot is translucent.

In the meantime, pulse the cashews in a food processor, just to chop them. Add the cooked shallot and garlic, and all of the remaining ingredients. Blend until smooth, scraping down the sides with a rubber spatula occasionally, to make sure you get everything. It may take 5 minutes or so to get it entirely smooth.

Keep the dressing refrigerated in a tightly sealed container until it's ready to use, for up to 5 days.

๑ INGREDIENT SCAVENGER HUNT

I love chanterelles in this because of their woodsy flavor and meaty texture. Problem is, they can be very hard to find out of season (or in season!). I would suggest any kind of fancy, wild mushroom such as maitake or trumpet. If you can't find those, either, then a thinly sliced portobello will totally suffice. ๑

Cool Slaw

SERVES 6 • ACTIVE TIME: 10 MINUTES • TOTAL TIME: 1 HOUR

PER SERVING
(⅙ RECIPE):
Calories: 60
Calories from fat: 25
Total fat: 2.5 g
Saturated fat: 0 g
Trans fat: 0 g
Total carb: 7 g
Fiber: 2 g
Sugars: 3 g
Protein: 2 g
Cholesterol: 0 mg
Sodium: 240 mg
Vitamin A: 40%
Vitamin C: 50%
Calcium: 4%
Iron: 4%

You know the phrase, "Cool as a cashew?" Of course you don't, I just made it up. But after tasting this recipe, you'll see why! A small handful of cashews make this coleslaw your coolest, creamiest, bestest friend. It's perfect to serve with BBQ or to cool down your **Buffalo Tempeh** (page 161).

DRESSING:

¼ cup cashew pieces

2 tablespoons chopped white onion

½ cup water

5 teaspoons apple cider vinegar

1 teaspoon Dijon mustard

1 teaspoon agave nectar

½ teaspoon salt

Freshly ground black pepper

1 (14-ounce) bag coleslaw mix

To make the dressing, place all its ingredients in a food processor. Blend for at least 5 minutes, using a rubber spatula to scrape down the sides often, until completely smooth. It's really important that you blend for the full time, otherwise your dressing may be grainy.

Pour the coleslaw mix into a mixing bowl. Add the dressing and mix well. Let it sit for at least 45 minutes, to get the cabbage nice and wilted so that it will absorb the dressing. Stir occasionally. Taste for salt and chill until ready to serve.

∾ TIPS

• If you've got time, soak the cashews in water for at least an hour or up to overnight. Drain the water and proceed with recipe. The soaking will make the cashews much easier to blend into smooth, creamy oblivion.

• The coleslaw will take to the dressing much faster if you let it wilt a bit beforehand. If you've got the time, just leave the coleslaw mix out at room temperature for a few hours before preparing the salad. ∾

Wild Rice Salad with Oranges & Roasted Beets

SERVES 4 • ACTIVE TIME: 15 MINUTES • TOTAL TIME: 15 MINUTES ONCE ALL INGREDIENTS ARE PREPARED, BUT MORE LIKE 2 HOURS IF NOT

This is a salad I enjoy a lot during the winter months, when beets are still abundant and citrus, although imported, is in season. This recipe is a cooking lesson unto itself—you'll learn a quick and yummy way to prepare roasted beets with no oil, how to create beautiful gems of orange segments, and how to toast sesame seeds. Making it once will give you a few skills that will last a lifetime and you will never have to read the recipe again.

1	navel orange
2	tablespoons sesame seeds
1	recipe **Orange–Sesame Vinaigrette** (recipe follows)
2	cups cooked wild rice, cooled
¼	cup dried currants
2	cups red leaf lettuce, torn into bite-size pieces
1	pound **Tinfoil Beets** (see box, page 40), cooled

First, prepare the orange segments. Slice a thin layer off the top and bottom of the orange, then place the orange right side up on the cutting board and simply slice the peel downward, using a chef's knife and following the natural curve of the orange. A little of the white part (called the pith) is okay; just try to get as much orange as you can. Then slice the orange widthwise and cut each piece into ¾-inch segments.

> ## ∾ INGREDIENT SCAVENGER HUNT
> *Wild rice has an alluring earthy flavor, but the price can be not so alluring. If your budget isn't feeling wild about it, go for a wild rice blend instead. That's got some long-grain brown rice thrown into the mix, but you still get that wild rice taste, texture, and color. ∾*

PER SERVING
(¼ RECIPE):
Calories: 230
Calories from fat: 50
Total fat: 6 g
Saturated fat: 1 g
Trans fat: 0 g
Total carb: 40 g
Fiber: 7 g
Sugars: 16 g
Protein: 7 g
Cholesterol: 0 mg
Sodium: 190 mg
Vitamin A: 25%
Vitamin C: 80%
Calcium: 6%
Iron: 10%

Then toast the sesame seeds. Preheat a small, heavy-bottomed pan over medium-low heat. Place the sesame seeds in the pan and stir often for about 2 minutes. They should be toasting by then (if not, then raise the heat). Use a spatula to toss continuously for another minute or so, until they are varying shades of toasty brown. Remove from the pan ASAP to prevent burning.

Pour the dressing into a large mixing bowl. Add the wild rice, currants, and lettuce. Using tongs, toss to coat. Add the orange segments and sesame seeds, and toss again. Last, fold in the beets. Serve.

Tinfoil Beets

Unwrapping a tinfoil beet is a lot like unwrapping a present. Well, maybe not really, because you know exactly what's going to be in there, but it's still somehow such an exciting surprise. Roasting brings out the beet's sweet flavor, so they're like precious rubies in a candy box when ready to eat. I usually do two pounds at a time on a weeknight or Sunday afternoon, and use some of them that evening as a side dish with whatever I'm eating. Then I refrigerate the rest and use them in salads or just for a quick snack throughout the week.

The cooking method and time really varies depending on the size of the beets you're using. If using small beets, say golf ball size, and they are very fresh, then don't bother to peel them first. Just slice in half, wrap in foil, and roast. And remember to save the beet greens to sauté with some olive oil and garlic. But if using those big honkers of a beet that you're more likely to find come January and February, then it's a little different. Peel them and then slice top down into segments (like orange slices) that are about ¾ inch thick at their widest. If a beet is especially big—say, softball size—then I sometimes will slice widthwise, too. Then, keeping all the slices together in a neat package, place on tinfoil and wrap so that you can easily unfold it from the top.

Roasting times will vary, but I do at least an hour at 425°F. They're ready when pierced easily with a fork. Be careful when handling, because there will be a lot of red beet juice just dying to drizzle out and stain your countertops. Although maybe that could look cool.

Orange-Sesame Vinaigrette

SERVES 4 • ACTIVE TIME: 10 MINUTES • TOTAL TIME: 10 MINUTES

This dressing is heavenly; fruity, toasty, spicy, and tangy. Toasted sesame oil is kind of a godsend for dressings because it has so much flavor and a little goes a long way.

¾ cup freshly squeezed orange juice (2 to 3 navel oranges)
2 tablespoons red wine vinegar
1 tablespoon toasted sesame oil
⅛ teaspoon salt
1 teaspoon hot chili sauce, such as Sriracha
1 teaspoon Microplaned or finely minced fresh ginger

Vigorously mix together all the ingredients. Just mix them right into a measuring cup so as not to use too many dishes. If you're using the dressing for a grain salad, you can also mix it directly into the large mixing bowl that you will use to prepare your salad. Keep refrigerated in a tightly sealed container until ready to use.

PER SERVING
(ABOUT ¼ CUP):
Calories: 50
Calories from fat: 30
Total fat: 3.5 g
Saturated fat: 0 g
Trans fat: 0 g
Total carb: 5 g
Fiber: 0 g
Sugars: 4 g
Protein: 0 g
Cholesterol: 0 mg
Sodium: 100 mg
Vitamin A: 0%
Vitamin C: 40%
Calcium: 0%

ɐ INGREDIENT SCAVENGER HUNT

Make sure your sesame oil is labeled "toasted sesame oil." Toasting the seeds brings out a lot of bold flavor, where regular sesame oil might just fall flat. It's usually found in the oil section of the supermarket, although sometimes it can be found in the Asian aisle. ɐ

Caesar Salad with Eggplant Bacon

SERVES 4 • ACTIVE TIME: 20 MINUTES • TOTAL TIME: 30 MINUTES

(CAN BE MADE GLUTEN FREE IF USING GF TAMARI IN PLACE OF SOY SAUCE)

Briny Caesar dressing meets smoky eggplant slices in this spin on the classic Caesar. I love all the texture going on, with the crunchy fresh romaine, creamy dressing, and the eggplant bacon—crisp in some places, chewy in others. To make this into more of an entrée salad, add some of **Basic Baked Tofu** (page 144) or a handful of chickpeas.

EGGPLANT BACON:

½   pound eggplant

2   tablespoons soy sauce

½   teaspoon liquid smoke

SALAD:

8   cups chopped romaine lettuce

1   recipe **Caesar Chavez Dressing** (recipe follows)

Preheat the oven to 425°F. Cover a large baking sheet with parchment paper.

Prep the eggplants while the oven is preheating. I slice them into half-moons because it's the easiest shape to slice consistently. Aim for eggplants that are around 4 inches in diameter at their widest. Cut off the stem and the bottom, then cut the eggplant in half lengthwise. Lay the eggplants halves cut side down, and cut into about ⅛-inch-thick slices. Don't worry if your slices are a bit irregular; that just adds to the texture, which should be varied between tender and chewy to smoky and crisp. What we're going to do is bake them at a high temperature with just a bit of nonstick cooking spray, then let them cool, then give them smoky salty flavor and reheat.

Place the eggplant strips in a single layer on the parchment paper. Spray lightly with cooking spray. Place in the oven and bake for about 8 minutes, keeping a close eye.

Remove the pan from the oven and flip the eggplant slices. They should be browning already, and if any are slightly burnt, don't worry. Just transfer them to a plate to let cool. Return the remaining slices to the oven for about 3 minutes.

Remove from the oven. The eggplant should be dark brown to burnt in some places, and yellowish white and tender in others. Transfer to a plate to let cool.

Lower the oven temperature to 350°F. When the eggplant is cool enough to handle, mix the soy sauce and liquid smoke together in a bowl. Dip the eggplant slices into the mixture and return them to the baking sheet. Bake for about 3 more minutes, until heated through. Serve within the next few hours.

Assemble the salad: Pour the dressing into a large mixing bowl. Add the lettuce in batches, using tongs to coat the lettuce after each addition. When all the lettuce is coated, transfer to bowls and top with eggplant bacon.

Caesar Chavez Dressing

SERVES 4 • ACTIVE TIME: 5 MINUTES • TOTAL TIME: 5 MINUTES

I am tempted to call this TaMiShew dressing, for the tahini, miso, and cashew in it, but I will spare you the cutesy title this time. But I won't spare you lots of flavor with a hint of brininess from the capers.

- 2 tablespoons chopped shallot
- 2 tablespoons cashew pieces
- 1 tablespoon tahini
- 1 tablespoon miso
- ⅓ cup water
- 2 tablespoons freshly squeezed lemon juice
- 1 teaspoon Dijon mustard
- 1 tablespoon capers with brine
- ⅛ teaspoon salt
  Freshly ground black pepper

PER SERVING (ABOUT 3 TABLESPOONS):
Calories: 60
Calories from fat: 40
Total fat: 4.5 g
Saturated fat: 0.5 g
Trans fat: 0 g
Total carb: 5 g
Fiber: <1 g
Sugars: <1 g
Protein: 2 g
Cholesterol: 0 mg
Sodium: 330 mg
Vitamin A: 0%
Vitamin C: 6%
Calcium: 0%
Iron: 4%

Place everything in a food processor and blend for at least 5 minutes, using a rubber spatula to scrape down the sides often, until completely smooth. It's really important that you blend for the full time, otherwise your dressing may be grainy. Taste for salt. Keep refrigerated in a tightly sealed container until ready to use.

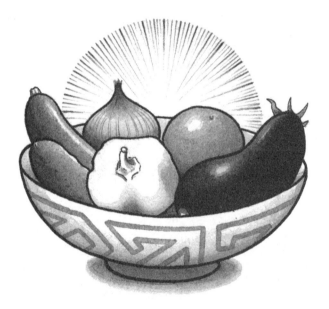

Vietnamese Rice Noodle Salad with Grilled Tofu

SERVES 6 • ACTIVE TIME: 30 MINUTES • TOTAL TIME: 40 MINUTES

(CAN BE MADE GLUTEN FREE IF USING GF TAMARI IN PLACE OF SOY SAUCE)

If cool and refreshing is how you like your salads, then this Vietnamese-inspired salad might be your true calling. Silky rice noodles, cool cucumbers, and refreshing mint are spiced up with some chili garlic sauce. I liked it best served with extra lime wedges and extra chili garlic sauce that you can spoon on to your liking. The grilled tofu is simply marinated in a little of the dressing to give it a little something. It's all sprinkled with a gremolata of peanut, mint, and lime for added flavor and texture. The directions look crazy long just because there are a few things going on, but it's not complicated.

DRESSING:

⅓ cup warm water

3 tablespoons agave nectar

3 tablespoons chili garlic sauce

1 tablespoon soy sauce

¼ cup freshly squeezed lime juice (about 2 limes, depending how juicy your limes are)

¼ teaspoon salt

SALAD:

12 ounces extra-firm tofu

2 teaspoons soy sauce

1 (8-ounce) package thin rice noodles (vermicelli)

1 medium-size cucumber, in thinly sliced half-moons (1 heaping cup, or 6 ounces)

1 small red onion, sliced thinly

4 ounces string beans, sliced into 1-inch pieces (about 1 cup)

2 cups mixed greens

¼ cup thinly sliced mint leaves

<hr>

PER SERVING
(⅙ RECIPE):
Calories: 260
Calories from fat: 60
Total fat: 7 g
Saturated fat: 1 g
Trans fat: 0 g
Fiber: 4 g
Protein: 10 g
Cholesterol: 0 mg
Sodium: 630 mg
Vitamin A: 8%
Vitamin C: 25%
Calcium: 20%
Iron: 15%

PEANUT-MINT GREMOLATA:

¼ cup peanuts, chopped very well

3 tablespoons finely chopped mint

Zest of ½ lime

To make the dressing, mix all its ingredients together and stir vigorously. Set aside.

Slice the tofu into eight equal pieces widthwise, then slice those rectangles corner to corner to form long triangles. Place in a single layer on a large plate and pour 6 tablespoons of the dressing over the slices. Also drizzle with 2 teaspoons of soy sauce. Let marinate, flipping occasionally, while you prepare everything else.

Cook the rice noodles according to the package directions. Usually they say to boil water, turn off the heat, and soak the noodles for about 8 minutes.

Once cooked, drain in a colander and run the noodles under cold water for about a minute until they are fully cooled. Set aside to drain while you finish prepping everything.

Mix all of the vegetables and the mint leaves into the noodles. Just use your hands—it's messy, but the best way I found to incorporate everything. Mix the dressing into the noodles and toss to coat. Refrigerate while you prepare everything else.

Combine the gremolata ingredients in a small bowl.

Now grill the tofu. Preheat a cast-iron grill or skillet over medium-high heat.

Spray the grill with nonstick cooking spray and grill the tofu on each side for about 4 minutes, or until grill marks appear. If using a pan, spray it with cooking spray and cook the tofu for 3 minutes on each side. Add the excess marinade to the noodles.

To serve: Scoop the noodles into six pretty bowls. Wedge two or three tofu pieces on the side of each bowl. Sprinkle with the gremolata and serve with lime wedges and extra chili garlic sauce.

> ⁓ TIP ⁓
>
> *To get the timing right, let me break it down:*
> - *Put on the water to boil.*
> - *Make the dressing, marinade the tofu.*
> - *Make the gremolata.*
> - *Cook the noodles.*
> - *Prep the veggies.*
> - *Drain the noodles.*
> - *Assemble the salad.*
> - *Grill the tofu.*
> - *Assemble the servings!*

Catalan Couscous Salad with Pears

SERVES 4 • ACTIVE TIME: 20 MINUTES • TOTAL TIME: 20 MINUTES

Inspired by Romesco sauce, the classic Catalan sauce of roasted red peppers and toasted nuts, this salad translation is divine tossed with whole wheat couscous and crisp, tart pears. Baby spinach adds some green and completes the scene. Toast the almonds for the dressing and the salad at the same time.

- ⅓ cup slivered almonds
- 2 cup cooked whole wheat couscous, cooled
- 4 cups baby spinach
- 1 thinly sliced Anjou pear (or any ripe pear)
- 1 recipe **Romesco Dressing** (recipe follows)

First toast the almonds. Preheat a small, heavy-bottomed pan over medium heat. Toss in the almonds and toast them, stirring often, for about 5 minutes. They should be varying shades of toasty brown and smell nutty and delicious.

In a large mixing bowl, toss together the couscous, spinach, and pears. Add the dressing and toss to coat. Divide among four plates and top with the toasted almonds.

PER SERVING
(¼ RECIPE):
Calories: 220
Calories from fat: 60
Total fat: 7 g
Saturated fat: 0.5 g
Trans fat: 0 g
Total carb: 32 g
Fiber: 6 g
Sugars: 6 g
Protein: 8 g
Cholesterol: 0 mg
Sodium: 520 mg
Vitamin A: 90%
Vitamin C: 90%
Calcium: 10%
Iron: 15%

Romesco Dressing

SERVES 4 • ACTIVE TIME: 10 MINUTES • TOTAL TIME: 10 MINUTES

You can't really go wrong with toasted almonds. I love the backdrop the almonds give this dressing; you can really taste them with every luscious bite.

PER SERVING
(¼ CUP):
Calories: 45
Calories from fat: 25
Total fat: 2.5 g
Saturated fat: 0 g
Trans fat: 0 g
Total carb: 4 g
Fiber: 1 g
Sugars: 2 g
Protein: 2 g
Cholesterol: 0 mg
Sodium: 470 mg
Vitamin A: 20%
Vitamin C: 60%
Calcium: 2%
Iron: 2%

3 tablespoons slivered almonds, toasted (see toasting directions, page 47)

2 tablespoons chopped shallot

¼ cup roasted red pepper from a jar, or 1 roasted red bell pepper, seeded and peeled (page 200)

½ cup water

3 tablespoons red wine vinegar

1 teaspoon Dijon mustard

½ teaspoon agave

¾ teaspoon salt

A few pinches of freshly ground black pepper

Pulse the almonds and shallot in a food processor, just to get them chopped up. Add the remaining ingredients and blend until relatively smooth. Taste for seasoning. Keep refrigerated and chilled in a tightly sealed container until ready to use, for up to 5 days.

Trattoria Pasta Salad with White Beans

SERVES 6 • ACTIVE TIME: 20 MINUTES • TOTAL TIME: 30 MINUTES

orget that tired old pasta salad Aunt Gertrude brings to the family reunions—this salad is where it's at! No mayo required. The Sun-dried Tomato–Walnut Dressing gives up plenty of flavor, beans keep you stuffed, and arugula gives you that trattoria feel. So tell Aunt Gertrude she's fired, but could she get you some freshly ground black pepper before she leaves? You can use jarred roasted red peppers or one red bell pepper you roast yourself.

- 8 ounces shell-shaped brown rice pasta
- 1 (15-ounce) can great northern beans, drained and rinsed
- 4 cups arugula
- 1 small red onion, sliced thinly
- ½ cup chopped roasted red pepper
- ¼ cup pitted kalamata olives, chopped in half
  Salt
  Freshly ground black pepper
- 1 recipe **Sun-dried Tomato–Walnut Dressing** (recipe follows)

First, cook the pasta al dente in salted water according to the package directions. Drain in a colander and rinse with cold water, then place in the fridge to cool completely.

Once the pasta has cooled, toss all the ingredients together in a large mixing bowl. Keep chilled until ready to eat.

> ∽ TIP *If it works out for your personal food plan for the day, throw ½ cup of toasted walnut halves into the mix.* ∽

PER SERVING
(⅙ RECIPE):
Calories: 290
Calories from fat: 45
Total fat: 5 g
Saturated fat: 0 g
Trans fat: 0 g
Total carb: 52 g
Fiber: 8 g
Sugars: 6 g
Protein: 10 g
Cholesterol: 0 mg
Sodium: 480 mg
Vitamin A: 15%
Vitamin C: 35%
Calcium: 8%
Iron: 15%
Option: ½ cup of toasted walnuts adds 65 calories, 6 grams of fat, 0.5 grams of saturated fat, and 1 gram of fiber.

Sun-dried Tomato–Walnut Dressing

SERVES 6 • ACTIVE TIME: 10 MINUTES • TOTAL TIME: 20 MINUTES

PER SERVING
(ABOUT 3
TABLESPOONS):
Calories: 40
Calories from fat: 20
Total fat: 2.5 g
Saturated fat: 0 g
Trans fat: 0 g
Total carb: 4 g
Fiber: <1 g
Sugars: 3 g
Protein: 1 g
Cholesterol: 0 mg
Sodium: 360 mg
Vitamin A: 0%
Vitamin C: 2%
Calcium: 0%
Iron: 2%

I love the zesty flavor of sun-dried tomatoes but don't love that they are usually packed in lots of oil. This dressing depends on walnuts instead of oil, and loose sun-dried tomatoes that are only packed in, well, air!

¼ cup sun-dried tomatoes (bought in dried form, not packed in oil)
3 tablespoons walnuts
½ teaspoon fennel seeds
2 tablespoons chopped shallot
¾ cup water
¼ cup balsamic vinegar
1 teaspoons Dijon mustard
¾ teaspoon salt
    A few pinches of freshly ground black pepper
½ teaspoon dried marjoram

First, rehydrate the tomatoes. Place them in a bowl and submerge in warm water. Let them soak for about 15 minutes, then drain.

Meanwhile, toast the walnuts. Preheat a small, heavy-bottomed pan over medium heat. Toss in the walnuts and toast them, stirring often, for about 7 minutes. They should be varying shades of toasty brown, and smell walnutty. Transfer immediately to a food processor.

Pulse the walnuts and fennel seeds to chop finely. Add the remaining ingredients, except for the marjoram, and puree until relatively smooth. Add the marjoram and pulse a few times to get it integrated. Keep the dressing refrigerated in a tightly sealed container for up to 5 days until ready to use.

Strawberry-Spinach Salad

MAKES 4 SERVINGS • ACTIVE TIME: 15 MINUTES • TOTAL TIME: 15 MINUTES

This is a simple and classic combination: sweet strawberries and earthy spinach, tied together by balsamic vinaigrette. It's the perfect summer salad! I love a little crunch in this salad, so the sunflower sprouts make a nice addition. You can also opt to add a tablespoon of toasted almonds to your serving, if you like. A package of baby spinach makes this super convenient, but the weight of the bags vary, so if yours is only 12 or 14 ounces, don't sweat it!

- 1   pound baby spinach leaves, washed well
- 1   pint strawberries, hulled and sliced thinly
- 1   recipe **Balsamic Vinaigrette** (page 17)
- 2   cups sunflower sprouts

In a large mixing bowl, combine the spinach, strawberries, and dressing. Toss together using tongs until well coated. Place on plates and top with sprouts. That's all she wrote.

PER SERVING
(¼ RECIPE):
Calories: 160
Calories from fat: 40
Total fat: 4.5 g
Saturated fat: 1 g
Trans fat: 0 g
Total carb: 26 g
Fiber: 4 g
Sugars: 10 g
Protein: 8 g
Cholesterol: 0 mg
Sodium: 590 mg
Vitamin A: 150%
Vitamin C: 140%
Calcium: 15%
Iron: 30%

Carrot-Ginger Dressing

MAKES 8 SERVINGS • ACTIVE TIME: 10 MINUTES • TOTAL TIME: 30 MINUTES

This is a great go-to dressing for a plain old garden salad. Add chickpeas, tofu . . . whatever you love in salad. I typically do red onion, fresh sliced mushrooms, tomato, cucumber . . . ya know, salad stuff. Boiling the carrots make them a flavorful, creamy, and colorful base for a dressing. I also love this as a thick sauce for a bowlful of steamed veggies, beans, and brown rice. It keeps well for at least 5 days, too. I don't get sick of it so I use it all week.

- ¾ pound carrots, peeled and sliced ½ inch thick
- 2 tablespoons chopped white onion
- 1 tablespoon minced fresh ginger
- 1 clove garlic
- ¼ cup freshly squeezed lime juice
- ¼ cup water, plus extra for thinning
- 1 tablespoon red wine vinegar
- 2 teaspoons toasted sesame oil
- 1 teaspoon light agave nectar
- ¼ teaspoon salt

First, we shall boil the carrots. Place them in a 2-quart pot and cover with water. Cover the pot and bring to a boil. Once boiling, lower the heat to a simmer and cook until the carrots are tender, about 15 minutes. Drain and run under cold water, then set aside.

Place the remaining ingredients in a food processor and pulse a few times to get the garlic chopped. Transfer the carrots to the food processor (it's okay if they're a bit warm). Blend until very smooth, scraping down.

CHAPTER 2

Totally Stuffed Sides

WHAT EXACTLY IS A SIDE DISH? WHEN EATING A PLANT-based diet, you're already kind of eating a diet comprised of what Americans *think* of as side dishes. So for the purposes of this book, sides are mostly grains and starchy, carby items that, with a little love, and maybe a few beans, can be miraculously transformed into main dishes. Side dishes don't need to be elaborate—in fact, oftentimes a scoop of plain old brown rice will get the job done. But these recipes are for when you want to go just a step beyond that.

Carbohydrates don't have to mean empty calories. Not in the least! Here you will find whole-grain dishes based on rice, quinoa, barley, and other grains that might be new to you, such as kasha, millet, and bulgur.

Also included here are comfort carbs, such as mashed potatoes cut with cauliflower, and sweet potatoes mashed with apple. Stuff that you wanna douse with gravy or barbecue sauce. Side dishes don't have to be thankless afterthoughts. Use this chapter when you want to dig in and get totally stuffed!

Cauliflower Mashed Potatoes (Caulipots)

SERVES 4 • ACTIVE TIME: 15 MINUTES • TOTAL TIME: 40 MINUTES

~~~~~~~~~~~~~~~

PER SERVING
(¼ RECIPE):
Calories: 190
Calories from fat: 35
Total fat: 3.5 g
Saturated fat: 0.5 g
Trans fat: 0 g
Total carb: 37 g
Fiber: 5 g
Sugars: 4 g
Protein: 6 g
Cholesterol: 0 mg
Sodium: 370 mg
Vitamin A: 0%
Vitamin C: 100%
Calcium: 4%
Iron: 10%

Mashed potatoes are pretty much the clouds of heaven—I definitely indulge—but the fat and calories therein can make them the spuds of hell. If the idea of life without mashed potatoes leaves you a shattered mess, Caulipots are there to pick up the pieces. With less than 200 calories per serving, they're perfect for those times when you want something much lighter. Serve 'em with something saucy and flavorful, such as the **Chickpea Piccata** (page 115) or **Portobello Pepper Steak Stew** (page 247), so that they can do their job of comfort starch most effectively.

> 2 russet potatoes, cut into ¾-inch pieces (about 1½ pounds)
> ½ head cauliflower, cut into florets (1 pound, or about 3 cups)
> 1 tablespoon olive oil
> 2 to 4 tablespoons vegetable broth
> ½ teaspoon salt
> Several pinches of freshly ground black pepper

Place the potatoes in a 4-quart pot in enough cold water to submerge them, making sure there are about 4 inches of extra water on top for when you add the cauliflower. Bring the potatoes to a boil. Once boiling, add the cauliflower and lower the heat to a simmer. Let simmer for about 15 minutes, until the potatoes and cauliflower are tender.

Drain them in a colander, return them to the pot, and use a potato masher to mash them a bit. Add the olive oil, 2 tablespoons of broth, and the salt and pepper, and mash a bit more. Use a fork to make sure all the seasonings are mixed well. If needed, add another 2 tablespoons of broth. Taste for salt. Serve warm.

A Trillion Ways to Dress Up Your Caulipots—or Maybe Just Six

Chipotle Caulipots: Remove the seeds from four canned chipotle peppers in adobe sauce. Finely mince and mix them into the Caulipots, along with 1 tablespoon of adobe sauce, or more to taste.

Garlic-Herb Caulipots: Mince four garlic cloves and sauté in the olive oil, along with 2 teaspoons of dried thyme and 1 teaspoon of dried marjoram. Mix into the mashed Caulipots.

Lemon-Dill Caulipots: Mix in 2 tablespoons of freshly squeezed lemon juice and 1 teaspoon of Microplaned lemon zest along with ¼ cup of finely chopped fresh dill.

Cheezy 'Pots: Add 3 tablespoons of nutritional yeast to the Caulipots.

Garden-Variety Caulipots: Sauté ¼ cup of chopped fresh chives and 2 tablespoons of chopped fresh flat-leaf parsley in the oil. Mix into the Caulipots. This is also fab with a hit of freshly squeezed lemon juice.

Broccopots: Replace the cauliflower with broccoli.

Silky Chickpea Gravy

SERVES 8 • ACTIVE TIME: 20 MINUTES • TOTAL TIME: 30 MINUTES

(CAN BE MADE GLUTEN FREE IF USING GF TAMARI IN PLACE OF SOY SAUCE)

~~~~~~~~~~~~~~~
PER SERVING
(⅛ RECIPE):
Calories: 70
Calories from fat: 15
Total fat: 1.5 g
Saturated fat: 0 g
Trans fat: 0 g
Total carb: 11 g
Sugars: 2 g
Fiber: 2 g
Protein: 3 g
Cholesterol: 0 mg
Sodium: 400 mg
Vitamin A: 0%
Vitamin C: 4%
Calcium: 2%
Iron: 6%

Gravy isn't exactly a "side," but what mashed potato recipe is complete without a gravy recipe? I really like to drown my food in gravy, so this tasty sauce comes in handy when I don't also want to drown my food in grease. Chickpeas give this gravy great body and a full, savory flavor. It's really a superhero that comes running when it hears the calls of potatoes from miles away, crying out for gravy.

1 teaspoon olive oil
1 small onion, chopped roughly
3 cloves garlic, chopped
2 teaspoons dried thyme
1 teaspoon dried rubbed sage (not powdered)
   Several pinches of freshly ground black pepper
2 tablespoons arrowroot powder
1¼ cups vegetable broth
1 (15-ounce) can chickpeas, drained and rinsed
2 tablespoons soy sauce or tamari (use wheat free for a gluten-free gravy)
   Salt

Preheat a saucepan over medium-high heat. Sauté the onion and garlic in the oil for about 5 minutes. Add the thyme, sage, and pepper, and cook for about 3 minutes more. While that is cooking, whisk the arrowroot into the veggie broth until dissolved.

If you have an immersion blender then add the beans, broth mixture, and soy sauce to the pot. Blend until smooth and lower the heat to medium, stirring often for about 10 minutes while it thickens.

If you are using a regular blender, place the broth mixture and beans in the blender and blend until smooth. Add the onions and other stuff from the pan to the blender and puree again until smooth. Add back to the pot and stir often over medium heat to thicken.

Once the gravy thickens, lower the heat to low. Now you can decide exactly how thick you want the gravy by adding splashes of water, anywhere between ¼ and ½ cup. Keep warm and covered until ready to serve.

Mashed Yuca with Cilantro & Lime

SERVES 6 • ACTIVE TIME: 10 MINUTES • TOTAL TIME: 40 MINUTES

I'm trying to think of ways to describe yuca in case you've never had it. What comes to mind is nutty, earthy, bitter, starchy . . . but that doesn't do this tropical root vegetable justice. Comparable to a potato when mashed, its flavor is more, as the French say, "I don't know what."

Because of how starchy yuca is, it's often mashed with a lot of oil. Instead, to get it creamy here, you'll reserve some of the boiling liquid and stream it back in as you mash. The yuca becomes creamy and ready to take on the sauce of whatever you're serving it with. Try something a little sweet, like **Mango BBQ Beans** (page 133) or the **Caribbean Curried Black-Eyed Peas with Plantains** (page 129). Some lime juice and cilantro finishes it off.

(page 133) (page 129)

- 2 pounds yuca, peeled and chopped into 2-inch chunks
- 2 tablespoons freshly squeezed lime juice
- ¼ cup chopped fresh cilantro
- 1 teaspoon olive oil
- ½ teaspoon salt, plus extra for salting the yuca water

> **TIP** Yuca usually comes with its outer peel waxed, to preserve freshness. That doesn't help you peel it, however! The easiest way I've found to peel yuca is to remove the rough ends and cut the yuca into thirds. Place a piece vertically on the cutting board, secure it with your nonwriting hand, and use a chef's knife to slice the skin off. If you don't have the best knife skills, a paring knife might work better but take a little longer. You might notice a fibrous core running down the center; slice that off once you've gotten the yuca into smaller pieces.

PER SERVING
(⅙ RECIPE):
Calories: 200
Calories from fat: 15
Total fat: 1.5 g
Saturated fat: 0 g
Trans fat: 0 g
Total carb: 45 g
Fiber: 2 g
Sugars: 0 g
Protein: 2 g
Cholesterol: 0 mg
Sodium: 210 mg
Vitamin A: 0%
Vitamin C: 50%
Calcium: 8%
Iron: 20%

Place the yuca in a pot and cover with water until submerged. Add a big pinch of salt, cover the pot, and bring to a boil. Lower the heat to a simmer. Let simmer for about 20 minutes, until very, very tender. Turn off the heat.

Reserve about a cup of the hot water by carefully dipping a heatproof mug into the pot. Don't burn yourself, please. Drain the yuca, then return it to the pot. Add the lime juice, cilantro, oil, and salt. Mash well with a potato masher. Stream in the reserved hot water little by little, mashing as you go along. You may need up to ½ cup. Mash the yuca until nice and creamy and serve immediately.

OMG Oven-Baked Onion Rings

SERVES 4 • ACTIVE TIME: 30 MINUTES • TOTAL TIME: 50 MINUTES

When my boyfriend requested low-fat onion rings, I kind of let out a sigh; maybe I even rolled my eyes. I'm not crazy about onion rings in the first place and so of course I would be even less crazy about low-fat ones. Right? Well, sometimes it feels good to be wrong! I ended up gaga over these. Somehow the greasy mess that is a diner onion ring became a thing of beauty when coated in some whole wheat bread crumbs and baked in a superhot oven.

PER SERVING
(¼ RECIPE)
Calories: 220
Calories from fat: 45
Total fat: 5 g
Saturated fat: 1 g
Trans fat: 0 g
Total carb: 38 g
Fiber: 3 g
Sugars: 5 g
Protein: 7 g
Cholesterol: 0 mg
Sodium: 520 mg
Vitamin A: 0%
Vitamin C: 10%
Calcium: 6%
Iron: 10%

- 2 Vidalia onions (about a pound), or other sweet onion such as Walla Walla
- ½ cup plus 2 tablespoons all-purpose flour
- 2 tablespoons cornstarch
- 1 cup cold almond milk
- 1 teaspoon apple cider vinegar
- 1 cup whole wheat bread crumbs
- 1 teaspoon kosher salt
- 2 teaspoons olive oil

Slice the onions into 3/4-inch-thick rings. Separate the rings and place in a bowl. Cover with a kitchen towel or something, to keep the onioniness out of your eyes.

Preheat the oven to 450°F. Line a rimmed 12 by 18-inch baking sheet with parchment paper, spray with cooking spray, and set aside.

Now you'll need two bowls for the batter and breading. If you've got large, wide cereal bowls, those'll do the trick. Into one bowl, dump the flour and cornstarch. Add about half of the almond milk and stir vigorously with a fork to dissolve. Add the rest of the almond milk and the apple cider vinegar, and stir to incorporate. Set aside.

In the other bowl, mix together the bread crumbs and salt. Drizzle in the oil and use your fingertips to mix it up well.

Get a conveyor belt going. From left to right, arrange the onions, the flour mixture, the bread-crumb mixture, and lastly the baking sheet. Dip each onion slice into the flour, letting the excess drip off. Transfer to the bread-crumbs bowl and use the other hand to sprinkle a handful of bread crumbs over the onion, to coat completely. This may take a bit of practice.

Carefully transfer each onion to a single layer on the baking sheet. Make sure you use one hand for the wet batter and the other for the dry batter, or you'll end up with club hand.

Spray the rings lightly with nonstick cooking spray and bake for 8 minutes. Flip, and bake for another 6 minutes. The rings should be varying shades of brown and crisp. Taste one to check for doneness. Serve as soon as possible. With ketchup if you must.

ᕦ COUPLA THINGS.

You have to use sweet onions for this. Otherwise the taste won't be as special and the texture won't be as juicy. Also, if things go as planned, you're not going to use all of the onions or all of the coating. Just use the nice big rings, and use the tiny inside rings for something else. For the batter and coating, you need a lot to get everything breaded, but there will be a bunch left over. Them's the breaks. ᕤ

Scallion Potato Pancakes

MAKES 6 SERVINGS, 2 PANCAKES EACH • ACTIVE TIME: 20 MINUTES • TOTAL TIME: 50 MINUTES

You know those super deep-fried Chinese takeout scallion pancakes? Those were my inspiration here. I wanted crispy and oniony and carby and satisfying. But I didn't want deep-fried and I didn't want tons of empty calories. These pancakes, made with potato, really filled the need. Panko makes them nice and crispy and a high baking temperature gets them nicely browned and gives them that satisfying scallion pancake pull.

Serve with the **Hoisin-Mustard Tofu** (page 153) and steamed broccoli or try the **Orange-Scented Broccoli** (page 100). Or for a snack, mix hot Chinese mustard with a hint of agave and dip away. They reheat wonderfully, so fridge the leftovers and satisfy your potato needs all week.

- 2 pounds Yukon Gold potatoes, peeled and cut into ¾-inch chunks
- 1½ cups thinly sliced scallions (from one bunch)
- 1½ teaspoons toasted sesame oil
- ½ teaspoon salt
- ½ teaspoon freshly ground black pepper
- ⅓ cup panko bread crumbs

BREADING:
- 1 cup panko bread crumbs
- ½ teaspoon salt
- ½ teaspoon freshly ground black pepper
- Cooking spray

PER SERVING
(2 PANCAKES):
Calories: 180
Calories from fat: 20
Total fat: 2.5 g
Saturated fat: 0 g
Trans fat: 0 g
Total carb: 35 g
Fiber: 4 g
Sugars: 2 g
Protein: 5 g
Cholesterol: 0 mg
Sodium: 430 mg
Vitamin A: 6%
Vitamin C: 60%
Calcium: 4%
Iron: 8%

> **TIP** *These are very delicate before being baked, so handle firmly but carefully when pressing into the bread crumbs and transferring to the pan. Once in the pan they will firm up nicely.*

First, boil the potatoes. Place them in a small pot and submerge in water. Cover and bring to a boil. Once boiling, lower the heat to a simmer and cook until tender, about 15 minutes.

Once cooked, run the potatoes under cold water. Let them cool for about 15 minutes, giving them a mix every now and again, until they are cool enough to handle.

Preheat the oven to 425°F. Line a large baking sheet with parchment paper and spray it with nonstick cooking spray. Place the potatoes in a mixing bowl and add the scallions, sesame oil, salt and black pepper. Use a potato masher to mash like crazy, until there aren't any big chunks of potato left. Add the panko and mix well.

ௗ NOTE *Because you need to use vegetable spray for these, I added 1 teaspoon of oil to the nutritional info.* ௐ

Mix together all of the breading ingredients on a large dinner plate. Form the pancakes by rolling ¼ cup of batter into a ball and then flattening it to a pancake about 4 inches in diameter. Press it firmly and carefully into the breading mixture, then transfer it to the prepared sheet. Bake in batches of six for best results.

When you have six pancakes on the sheet and the oven is preheated, spray the pancakes lightly with cooking spray. Place in the oven and bake for 12 minutes. Flip carefully, using a thin spatula, and spray the pancakes on the other side. Bake for 8 more minutes.

They're best when served warm!

Ginger Mashed Sweet Potatoes & Apples

SERVES 6 • ACTIVE TIME: 20 MINUTES • TOTAL TIME: 50 MINUTES

For me there is no better comfort food than sweet potatoes. Warm, sweet, creamy, and spicy, what more could you want? Something bright orange? Well, this dish has you covered. The apples brighten everything up and give the sweet potatoes an air of mystery. In the autumn months this makes such a flavorful and simple base for myriad stews, or just serve with baked tofu or tempeh and greens. And it's virtually fat free! I'm the queen of hating to peel things, but it really makes everything so much creamier and yummier. It's nice to have uninterrupted mushiness, so take the trouble to peel your apples and sweet potatoes here.

> 1 pound apples (2 average-size), peeled and cut into ½-inch chunks
> 2 pounds sweet potatoes or yams, peeled and cut into ½-inch chunks
> ¼ cup water
> ¼ teaspoon salt
> 1 tablespoon agave (optional; see note)
> ¼ teaspoon ground cinnamon
> ½ teaspoon grated fresh ginger (see tip)

PER SERVING (⅙ RECIPE):
Calories: 180
Calories from fat: 0
Total fat: 0 g
Saturated fat: 0 g
Trans fat: 0 g
Total carb: 44 g
Fiber: 7 g
Sugars: 16 g
Protein: 3 g
Cholesterol: 0 mg
Sodium: 180 mg
Vitamin A: 430%
Vitamin C: 15%
Calcium: 8%
Iron: 6%

Preheat a 4-quart pot over low heat. Spray it with nonstick cooking spray, then add the apples, sweet potatoes, water, and salt. Cover the pot and sweat the apples and sweet potatoes for about 20 minutes, stirring often. What this means is just to cook them slowly and let them steam. You want to coax the moisture out of them, but if you set the flame too high they'll burn and cook unevenly.

> ∽ **NOTE** I love to use sweet red apples in this. Fuji, McIntosh, or Rome would be perfect. Depending on how sweet your apples are, you may need even less agave than listed, or perhaps even no agave at all! Taste before adding. ∽

After 20 minutes, you can turn up the heat just a bit. Add a little more water if needed. Cover and cook for 20 more minutes, paying close attention so that they don't burn, and stirring often. When they're very tender, they're done. Mash with a potato masher. Add the agave, cinnamon, and ginger, and mash some more. Taste for salt and seasoning. Serve warm.

∾ TIPS

• Ginger can be daunting, navigating all those curves and nubs. So instead of letting the thought of ginger dissuade you from cooking dinner, try this. The second you get home from grocery shopping, or at least as soon as your ice cream is in the freezer, peel the ginger with a spoon. Take a teaspoon and scrape its side, face down, against the ginger skin. The skin peels right off and the spoon breezes over the nubby curves. If there is too much of a nub I just slice it off and sacrifice it or use it for tea.

• Once peeled, chop the ginger into manageable pieces, put it in a plastic bag, and freeze. For this dish, you don't even need to let it thaw because frozen ginger grates perfectly in this recipe. If you do want the ginger thawed, let it sit in the fridge all day. If not, briefly run a piece under hot water. Then proceed as usual. It really saves a lot of time! ∾

Brussels Sprout–Potato Hash

SERVES 4 • ACTIVE TIME: 30 MINUTES • TOTAL TIME: 45 MINUTES

The perfect breakfast for vegan lumberjacks! Making hash traditionally involves chopping up a bunch of stuff you have hanging
out around the house and pan-frying it until crispy. One day I had
a handful of Brussels sprouts, so they were the morning's hash victim,
and I loved it so much I put the recipe into permanent rotation. They're
flavored with thyme and lemon, my favorite morning blend. I call for
Yukon Golds here, but any thin-skinned potato will do. Serve with
scrambled tofu or make it a Benedict, with a sliced portobello on top and
some cheezy sauce. They'd also be none too bad with some **Silky Chickpea Gravy** (page 56).

PER SERVING
(¼ RECIPE):
Calories: 150
Calories from fat: 25
Total fat: 2.5 g
Saturated fat: 0 g
Trans fat: 0 g
Total carb: 29 g
Fiber: 4 g
Sugars: 3 g
Protein: 5 g
Cholesterol: 0 mg
Sodium: 600 mg
Vitamin A: 8%
Vitamin C: 100%
Calcium: 6%
Iron: 10%

- 2 teaspoons olive oil
- ½ pound Brussels sprouts, quartered lengthwise
- 1 pound Yukon Gold potatoes, cut into ½-inch pieces
- 1 small onion, diced small
- 3 cloves garlic, minced
- 2 teaspoons dried thyme
  Freshly ground black pepper
- 1 teaspoon salt
- 2 teaspoons grated lemon zest (zest from 1 lemon)

Preheat a large, heavy pan, preferably cast iron, over medium heat. Sauté
the potatoes and sprouts in 1 teaspoon of the oil, using nonstick cooking spray as necessary. Cover the pan and cook for about 30 minutes,
stirring occasionally, until the potatoes are tender and lightly browned.
Add the onion, garlic, thyme, pepper, salt, and lemon zest. Drizzle with
the remaining teaspoon of oil. Cook for another 15 minutes, stirring occasionally, until the onions are browned. Serve!

Polenta Stuffing

SERVES 4 • ACTIVE TIME: 10 MINUTES • TOTAL TIME: 30 MINUTES

I first discovered polenta stuffing when I was writing my dissertation on what to do with leftover polenta. Well, while it was being peer reviewed I had some time to reflect on the fact that store-bought polenta could be pretty handy at times, too. Especially if you're looking for a speedy weeknight side dish. So if you don't have any leftover polenta, no shame on you, just grab one of those tubes from the supermarket—many of them are fat free. If you love corn bread stuffing, I think you'll love polenta stuffing even more. It gets crispy on the outside with a comforting mushy interior and has all those herby stuffing tastes of thyme, celery, and sage. Because the serving is kind of small, I like to serve it on top of my main dish instead of on the side, such as the **Tamarind BBQ Tempeh & Sweet Potatoes** (page 159).

  2 teaspoons olive oil
18 ounces prepared polenta, cut into ¾-inch cubes (3½ cups)
½ cup thinly sliced celery
  1 small onion, cut into ½-inch dice
  2 cloves garlic, minced
¼ teaspoon dried sage
½ teaspoon dried thyme
    Freshly ground black pepper
½ teaspoon salt

Preheat a large pan, preferably cast iron, over medium-high heat. Pour in 1 teaspoon of the oil and coat the bottom of the pan. Sauté the polenta for 12 to 15 minutes, flipping often, until the outsides are lightly browned. Use some nonstick cooking spray to help you out a bit.

    Mix in the celery, onion, garlic, sage, thyme, and pepper, drizzle with the remaining oil, and sprinkle with salt. Sauté for another 7 to 10 minutes, until the onions are browned.

Cranberry-Cashew Biryani

SERVES 4 • ACTIVE TIME: 20 MINUTES • TOTAL TIME: 1 HOUR

I know that 95 percent of you won't care, but for all you astute foodies or Indian food experts, I know that this isn't officially a biryani. It's more of a pilaf because it's all cooked in one pot. I called it a biryani, though, because it's inspired by that Indian restaurant staple rice dish with the pretty yellow hue, brimming with fruits, nuts, and veggies. I used dried cranberries here, which provide a really nice burst of tartness.

If you can find the crannies sweetened with orange juice, then awesome. If not and you don't want added sugar, then plain old raisins will be just great. Cashew "pieces" are often sold in bulk at a lower price than whole cashews, which is so silly but a good deal for us. If you can't find them, then just roughly chop the cashews before adding them. Serve with **Eggplant–Chickpea Curry** (page 230) or any of the Indian curries.

PER SERVING
(¼ RECIPE):
Calories: 290
Calories from fat: 50
Total fat: 6 g
Saturated fat: 1 g
Trans fat: 0 g
Total carb: 54 g
Fiber: 4 g
Sugars: 8 g
Protein: 7 g
Cholesterol: 0 mg
Sodium: 360 mg
Vitamin A: 110%
Vitamin C: 10%
Calcium: 6%
Iron: 15%

    1   teaspoon vegetable oil
    1   teaspoon cumin seeds
    1   teaspoon mustard seeds
    3   cloves garlic, minced
    1   cup small-diced carrots
    1   cup brown jasmine or basmati rice
    1   teaspoon garam masala
    ¼   teaspoon turmeric
    ¼   teaspoon red pepper flakes
    ½   teaspoon salt
  2½   cups water
    1   tablespoon tomato paste
    ¼   cup dried cranberries
    ¼   cup roasted cashew pieces
    ½   cup frozen peas
        Chopped fresh cilantro, for garnish (optional)

Preheat a 2-quart pot over medium heat. Pour the oil into the pot and mix in the cumin and mustard seeds. Cover the pot and let the seeds pop for about a minute, or until the popping slows down, mixing once. If the seeds don't pop, turn up the heat a bit until they do.

Add the garlic and sauté for about a minute. Add the carrots, rice, garam masala, turmeric, red pepper flakes, and salt, and stir constantly for about a minute. Add the water and tomato paste. Cover and bring to a boil. Once boiling, lower the heat as low as it will go and cook, covered, for about 40 minutes.

After 40 minutes the water should be mostly absorbed. Stir in the cranberries, cashews, and peas. Cook for another 15 minutes or so, until the water is completely absorbed. Fluff the rice with a fork and serve topped with the cilantro, if using.

∽ NUTRITION TIP

Cashews and other nuts get a bad rap 'cause of the fat content, but much of it is healthy monounsaturated fat. And they are naturally high in trace minerals, such as zinc. Zinc is required for growth and development and a healthy immune system. If you are mindful of portion sizes, nuts can fit into a healthy diet. ∽

Scarlet Barley

SERVES 6 • ACTIVE TIME: 20 MINUTES • TOTAL TIME: 50 MINUTES

A fun and beautiful way to get those beets in. If you're going through the rice and quinoa humdrums, then barley is a great change of pace. With its satisfying, chewy texture and earthy flavor, it might be just what the doctor (or nutritionist) ordered. Serve with something that's also super earthy and flavorful, such as **Mushroom & Cannellini Paprikas** (page 127).

PER SERVING
(⅙ RECIPE):
Calories: 160
Calories from fat: 10
Total fat: 1.5 g
Saturated fat: 0 g
Trans fat: 0 g
Total carb: 33 g
Fiber: 7 g
Sugars: 5 g
Protein: 5 g
Cholesterol: 0 mg
Sodium: 370 mg
Vitamin A: 0%
Vitamin C: 15%
Calcium: 4%
Iron: 8%

1   teaspoon olive oil
2   cloves garlic, minced
    Freshly ground black pepper
1   bay leaf
1   cup pearl barley, rinsed
2½ cups vegetable broth
¼   teaspoon salt
1   beet (about ¾ pound), grated
    Juice of ½ lemon
    Fresh dill, for garnish (optional)

Preheat a 2-quart pot over medium heat. Sauté the garlic in the olive oil for about 30 seconds. Add several pinches of pepper and the bay leaf. Add the barley, broth, and salt; cover and bring to a boil. Once boiling, stir and lower the heat to low. Cover and cook for about 20 minutes, stirring occasionally.

When most of the water has absorbed, mix in the grated beet. Cook for about 20 more minutes, stirring occasionally. Turn off the heat, mix in the lemon juice, and taste for salt. Cover and let sit for about 10 more minutes. Remove the bay leaf and serve topped with fresh dill.

Unfried Fried Rice

4 SERVINGS • ACTIVE TIME: 15 MINUTES • TOTAL TIME: 1 HOUR, 15 MINUTES

(CAN BE MADE GLUTEN FREE IF USING GF TAMARI IN PLACE OF SOY SAUCE)

PER SERVING
(¼ RECIPE):
Calories: 260
Calories from fat: 25
Total fat: 3 g
Saturated fat: 0.5 g
Trans fat: 0 g
Total carb: 51 g
Fiber: 6 g
Sugars: 5 g
Protein: 8 g
Cholesterol: 0 mg
Sodium: 420 mg
Vitamin A: 130%
Vitamin C: 80%
Calcium: 6%
Iron: 15%

Fried rice is, well, really *fried*! This version tastes lighter, fresher, and delicious in its own right. Shallot, ginger, garlic, and green onion are all simple flavors that go a long way. Serve with **Hoisin-Mustard Tofu** (page 153) or any Chinese-inspired feast. The reason it takes so long is because the rice needs to cool a bit before you sauté it, but it's really an easy recipe. To make it ridiculously easy, make the rice a day ahead. In fact, refrigerated rice gives fried rice the perfect texture, so it's even preferable to do it that way.

    1   cup brown basmati or jasmine rice
    2   cups water
    1   teaspoon sesame oil
    ⅓   cup minced shallot
    3   cloves garlic, minced
    2   teaspoons minced fresh ginger
    1   tablespoon plus 1 teaspoon soy sauce
    ½   cup finely chopped green onion

First, cook the rice as you normally would. I use a small enameled cast-iron pot with a cover, bring the rice and water to a boil, then lower the heat to as low as it will go and cook for about 35 minutes. Once most of the water has been absorbed, turn off the heat and keep the rice covered for 15 more minutes.

Transfer the rice to a baking pan and spread it out to make it cool faster. If it's still steaming when you add it to the pan in the next step, it might get mushy.

Preheat a skillet over medium heat. Sauté the shallot, garlic, and ginger in the sesame oil for about 2 minutes. Add the rice and drizzle in the soy sauce. Toss to coat completely and cook for about 3 more minutes, until the rice is uniformly browned. Stir in the green onion and serve.

Variations:

This recipe is the very barest of bones, but you can add almost any veggie to bulk it up. A few ideas for ingredients to add a minute before you add the rice:

1 cup broccoli florets, steamed for 5 minutes
1 cup zucchini, diced into $\frac{1}{3}$-inch pieces, steamed for 5 minutes
1 cup carrot, diced into $\frac{1}{3}$-inch pieces, steamed for 7 minutes
1 cup frozen peas (thawed)
1 cup snow peas

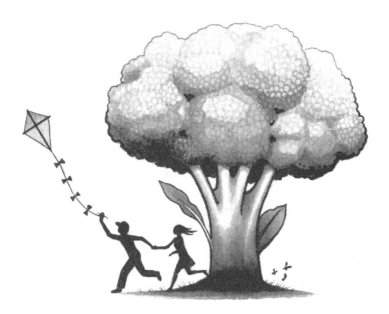

Bhutanese Pineapple Rice

SERVES 4 • ACTIVE TIME: 15 MINUTES • TOTAL TIME: 1 HOUR

(CAN BE MADE GLUTEN FREE IF USING GF TAMARI IN PLACE OF SOY SAUCE)

~~~~~~~~~~~~~~~~~~
PER SERVING
(¼ RECIPE):
Calories: 230
Calories from fat: 15
Total fat: 2 g
Saturated fat: 0 g
Trans fat: 0 g
Total carb: 49 g
Fiber: 3 g
Sugars: 8 g
Protein: 5 g
Cholesterol: 0 mg
Sodium: 430 mg
Vitamin A: 8%
Vitamin C: 50%
Calcium: 6%
Iron: 8%

I love Bhutanese red rice here for the firm and flavorful and dare I say toothsome texture. It almost seems like it's fried! Instead it's just a way healthy and damn pretty whole-grain rice. If you can't find this particular rice, brown jasmine or basmati will do.

1 cup Bhutanese red rice, prepared per package directions
1 teaspoon olive oil
1 small red onion, diced small
4 cloves garlic, minced
1 tablespoon minced ginger
Pinch of salt
2 teaspoons Thai red curry paste
1 tablespoon water
1 tablespoon soy sauce
2 teaspoons agave nectar
½ cup lightly packed fresh cilantro, chopped, plus extra for garnish
1½ cups diced pineapple (about ½-inch dice)

Preheat a skillet over medium heat. Sauté the onion, garlic, and ginger in the oil with a pinch of salt for about 5 minutes, until the onion is translucent. Meanwhile, in a small bowl, mix together the curry paste, water, soy sauce, and agave.

Add the cilantro to the skillet and sauté just until wilted, about a minute. Add the cooked rice and drizzle in the curry paste mixture. Toss to coat completely and cook for about 3 more minutes. Add the pineapple and cook just until heated through. Serve garnished with extra cilantro.

Sautéed Kasha & Mushrooms with Dill

SERVES 4 • ACTIVE TIME: 15 MINUTES • TOTAL TIME: 45 MINUTES

Y ou might know this dish as Kasha Varnishkes or you might be from western Nebraska and have no idea what I'm talking about. Either way, I can't imagine kasha without mushrooms. Maybe in a knish, but that's it! If I am going to make kasha, I am going to sauté some onions and mushrooms, too, and that's just the way it is. Kasha has such an assertive flavor that you really don't need much else; a little sweetness from the onion, a little earthiness from the mushroom, and a little herbiness from the dill.

Serve this with some baked tempeh and greens, if you like. I often just eat a double serving as my dinner because I find it addicting. You'll notice I use 2 teaspoons of oil here, and for this book that's a lot, but I really do like to get the onion nice and brown or it doesn't taste right to me. Two teaspoons does the trick!

1 cup coarse kasha, picked over and rinsed
2 cups water
2 teaspoons olive oil
1 medium-size onion, quartered and sliced thinly
½ teaspoon salt, plus a pinch for the kasha pot
1 pound cremini mushrooms, sliced
  Freshly ground black pepper
¼ cup chopped fresh dill

PER SERVING
(¼ RECIPE):
Calories: 210
Calories from fat: 35
Total fat: 3.5 g
Saturated fat: 0.5 g
Trans fat: 0 g
Total carb: 40 g
Fiber: 6 g
Sugars: 4 g
Protein: 9 g
Cholesterol: 0 mg
Sodium: 310 mg
Vitamin A: 4%
Vitamin C: 6%
Calcium: 8%
Iron: 15%

∾ INGREDIENT SCAVENGER HUNT

Kasha is toasted buckwheat groats, which is not actually wheat. It is in fact from a weird little plant that is in a class by itself and it's completely gluten free! It might be relegated to the "ethnic" section of your supermarket, or it might be by the rice. A popular brand is Wolf's, in a little black box. ∾

In a heavy-bottomed 2-quart pot, cover and bring the kasha, water, and big pinch of salt to a boil. Once boiling, lower the heat to a simmer and cook for about 15 minutes, stirring occasionally, until the kasha is tender. Remove from the heat.

Preheat a large nonstick skillet over medium heat. Sauté the onion for 7 to 10 minutes, until browned. Sprinkle with the ½ teaspoon of salt a few minutes into cooking, to draw out the moisture. Add the mushrooms and pepper. Sauté until tender and lightly browned, about 7 minutes. Add the kasha and toss to mix well. Toss in the dill, taste for seasoning, and serve.

> ∾ **TIP** *A really supergreat idea is to make the kasha in the morning. If you take an hour to get ready for work or whatever, why not have some kasha cooking on the stove? It ain't no thing! Then just pop it into the fridge, and when you're ready to make this dish, it will only take 20 minutes or so. And truth be told, it comes out better when the kasha has had a chance to chill. ∾*

Quinoa Puttanesca

SERVES 4 • ACTIVE TIME: 20 MINUTES • TOTAL TIME: 30 MINUTES

I'm always on the lookout for ways to incorporate quinoa and other grains into my meals, so it's pretty brainless to just make a traditional pasta sauce and toss it on a grain instead. If you're anything like me, you always have a gigantic thing of capers and olives in your fridge (not to mention great bone structure and an impressive unicorn collection.) Puttanesca is a really quick way to put together a complex-tasting—passionate, even—dish with pantry staples. Its ingredients and method are simple enough that you can prep it, cook it, and clean up after yourself in a leisurely 30 minutes, and then get back to the matter at hand. Succulent, salty, and a little spicy, this is in the "sides" section, but really, it makes a great dinner on its own.

PER SERVING
(¼ RECIPE):
Calories: 230
Calories from fat: 60
Total fat: 7 g
Saturated fat: 0.5 g
Trans fat: 0 g
Fiber: 8 g
Protein: 8 g
Cholesterol: 0 mg
Sodium: 930 mg
Vitamin A: 30%
Vitamin C: 35%
Calcium: 10%
Iron: 25%

2   cups cooked quinoa

SAUCE:
2   teaspoons olive oil
4   cloves garlic, chopped
1   teaspoon dried thyme
1   teaspoon crushed red pepper flakes
    A generous pinch of dried tarragon
    A generous pinch of dried marjoram
¼   cup white wine
½   cup kalamata olives, chopped roughly (sliced in half is great, too)
½   cup capers
1   (28-ounce) can crushed tomatoes
    Freshly ground black pepper

Preheat a saucepot over medium heat. Place the oil and garlic in the pot and stir for about a minute, being careful not to burn the garlic. Add the herbs, spices, and wine; cook for about a minute.

Add the olives, capers, and tomatoes. Cook for about 15 minutes.

You can serve by scooping quinoa into individual bowls and pouring the sauce over it, but my way is to just mix everything into a bowl together and reserve a little sauce to pour over my serving, because I like it extra hors d'oeuvre-y.

> ∾ TIP   I like to make a big batch of quinoa at the beginning of the week and store it for a few days. If you don't have a few cups of cooked quinoa around, then start your quinoa before starting your sauce: Mix 1 cup of uncooked quinoa with 2 cups water, bring to a boil, then lower the heat and cook uncovered for about 15 minutes, stirring occasionally, until the grain is tender and the water has been absorbed. ∾

Soft Broccoli Polenta

SERVES 6 • ACTIVE TIME: 30 MINUTES • TOTAL TIME: 30 MINUTES

Polenta is a fabulous side on its own—creamy, comforting, and oh-so-healthy for you! I'm very particular about how I eat my soft polenta, first running my spoon around the edges where it's cooled down a bit. I love to smother it in saucy beans or veggies and its luscious corn flavor goes with so many types of cuisine. Go Italian with **Chickpea Piccata** (page 115), or **Mexican with the Black Beans in Red Velvet Mole** (page 134). Barbecue works, too, so try it with the **Tamarind BBQ Tempeh & Sweet Potatoes** (page 159). Finely chopped broccoli is my favorite polenta add-in, for its texture and gardeny flavor. It just *feels* good to eat a bowlful of polenta!

> 4 cups vegetable broth
> ½ teaspoon salt, plus more to taste
> 1 cup polenta corn grits (polenta)
> 4 cups very well-chopped broccoli stalks and tops
> A few pinches of freshly ground black pepper

In a 2-quart saucepot, bring the water and the ½ teaspoon of salt to a boil. Add the polenta in a slow steady stream, whisking contantly as you pour it in. Add the broccoli and turn the heat down low. Let cook for 15 minutes, stirring often. Turn off the heat and cover, let sit for 10 more minutes, stirring occasionally. Serve hot!

PER SERVING
(⅙ RECIPE):
Calories: 120
Calories from fat: 5
Total fat: 0.5 g
Saturated fat: 0 g
Trans fat: 0 g
Total carb: 24 g
Fiber: 2 g
Sugars: 2 g
Protein: 4 g
Cholesterol: 0 mg
Sodium: 580 mg
Vitamin A: 10%
Vitamin C: 90%
Calcium: 4%
Iron: 8%

Ethiopian Millet

SERVES 4 • ACTIVE TIME: 15 MINUTES • TOTAL TIME: 45 MINUTES

Millet is like a blank slate, making it a perfect vehicle for spicy Ethiopian flavors. This dish goes perfectly with the **Mushroom Tibs** (page 95), as they have essentially the same flavor profile.

1 cup millet, rinsed and drained
2 cups water
1 teaspoon olive oil
1 small onion, diced small
3 cloves garlic, minced
1 tablespoon minced fresh ginger
½ teaspoon red pepper flakes
½ teaspoon salt
  Freshly ground black pepper
2 plum tomatoes, chopped
2 teaspoons curry powder
2 teaspoons Hungarian paprika
2 teaspoons ground cumin
¼ teaspoon ground cardamom
⅛ teaspoon ground cloves
2 to 4 tablespoons vegetable broth

First, prepare the millet. Place the millet in a 2-quart pot and cover with 2 cups of water. Cover and bring to a boil, then give it a stir and bring the heat down to very low. Cook, covered, for another 15 minutes or so, or until the water has been absorbed and the millet is fluffy. Turn off the heat, but keep the millet covered until ready to add to the pan.

While the millet is cooking, preheat a large skillet over medium heat. Sauté the onion, garlic, and ginger in the oil for about 5 minutes, until the onion is translucent. Add the red pepper flakes, salt, black pepper, and tomatoes, and sauté for about 2 minutes to break down the tomatoes a bit. Add the remainder of the spices, cover, and cook for 5 more minutes to further break down the tomatoes.

Add the millet to the pan and stir, and cook for 5 more minutes. Add the vegetable broth if things appear too dry. Taste for salt and spices, and serve.

All Vegans Have a Pleather Costanza Wallet

You know that *Seinfeld* episode where George's wallet is so fat he can't even close it? Well, that's exactly how us vegans are, but our wallets are stuffed with dollar bills from all the money we save! Many vegans know that bulk bins are the way to go. And I don't mean graze the bulk bins and eat free cashews. I mean buy your food in bulk and save some serious cash. Buying in bulk doesn't mean you have to buy bushels at a time, just exactly what you need so nothing goes to waste. Grains, spices, and nuts are all perfect bulk bin-purchase candidates.

Butternut Coconut Rice

SERVES 6 • ACTIVE TIME: 20 MINUTES • TOTAL TIME: 1½ HOURS

How can one rice dish be so much to so many? Savory, spicy, creamy, tangy, and slightly sweet—this recipe has got it all. Plus it's a gorgeous orange color! I'm not crazy about peeling butternut squash (who is?) and so I roast it in the oven, thus the long cooking time with lots of downtime. Try it; you'll see how convenient it is! Just roast away while the rice is cooking; it should take about the same time and once that's done everything will come together in a snap.

I love the aroma of brown basmati rice here, but you can use whatever rice you like best. Serve with **Pineapple Collards** (page 93) and **Broiled Blackened Tofu** (page 147).

1 cup brown basmati rice

2 cups water

A pinch of salt

2 pounds butternut squash

2 teaspoons sesame oil

1 cup sliced shallot

1 tablespoon minced fresh ginger

3 cloves garlic, minced

1 teaspoon lime zest

¼ teaspoon red pepper flakes

¼ teaspoon salt

¾ cup light coconut milk

¼ to ½ cup vegetable broth

1 tablespoon freshly squeezed lime juice

First, preheat the oven to 400°F (for the squash) and cook your rice according to the package directions, or however you prefer to cook rice. I rinse the rice and then add it to a 2-quart pot along with the water and a pinch of salt. Cover and bring to a boil. Once boiling, immediately lower the heat as low as it will go and cook for about an hour.

For the squash, slice off the bulbous part. Slice in half lengthwise, exposing the seeds. Scoop the seeds out with a tablespoon. Slice the long part of the squash in half lengthwise as well. Line a baking sheet with parchment paper and place the squash face down on the sheet. Bake for about 45 minutes. Once it's soft enough to pierce with a fork, remove it from the oven and let it cool. (Place it outside to cool if possible; that'll speed things up.) When the squash is cool enough to handle, proceed with the recipe.

Preheat a large skillet over medium heat. Sauté the shallot in the oil, using a little nonstick cooking spray if needed, until lightly browned, about 7 minutes. Add the ginger, garlic, lime zest, red pepper flakes, and salt, and sauté for another 2 minutes. Turn down the heat to low.

Scoop the flesh out of the squash and add it to the pan, along with the coconut milk. Use a potato masher (or a fork) to mash the butternut into a creamy consistency. Add the rice and stir well. Add ¼ cup of the vegetable broth and mix well. You can add up to another ¼ cup of broth to get a creamier consistency if you like. Add the lime juice, taste for salt, and serve!

> ∾ TIP *If you want a little more coconutty goodness, you can add a tablespoon of toasted coconut to each finished serving. It lends lots of flavor and texture, if you have some extra time and calories burning a hole in your pocket.*
>
> *To toast coconut, preheat a large pan over low heat and place 6 tablespoons of shredded (unsweetened!) coconut in the pan. Stir often. The coconut will start to toast and turn a few shades darker. It should take about 5 minutes. Remove from the heat immediately.* ∾

Eggplant Kibbeh

SERVES 6 • ACTIVE TIME: 25 MINUTES • TOTAL TIME: 1 HOUR 15 MINUTES

PER SERVING
(⅙ RECIPE):
Calories: 130
Calories from fat: 15
Total fat: 1.5 g
Saturated fat: 0 g
Trans fat: 0 g
Total carb: 28 g
Fiber: 9 g
Sugars: 4 g
Protein: 5 g
Cholesterol: 0 mg
Sodium: 400 mg
Vitamin A: 15%
Vitamin C: 20%
Calcium: 6%
Iron: 10%

If you look up *kibbeh* in Wikipedia, you'll find a million different variations, shapes, and definitions. But perhaps you aren't a nerd who immediately looks things up on Wikipedia and then doubts its validity, so I will just tell you this: kibbeh, as I know it, is a Lebanese dish of bulgur, mixed with usually mushy veggies (the vegan versions of kibbeh, at least), spices, and mint. It goes fabulously with a Mediterranean meze, so break out the hummus for this one.

1 cup bulgur, rinsed and drained
1 teaspoon olive oil
1 small onion, diced finely
4 cloves garlic, minced
1 pound eggplant, cut into ½-inch pieces
1 teaspoon salt
  Freshly ground black pepper
3 plum tomatoes, chopped
2 teaspoons ground cumin
½ cup fresh chopped mint, plus extra for garnish

First, prepare the bulgur. Boil 1⅓ cups of water in a kettle. Place the bulgur in a small pot that has a secure-fitting lid; I have a 2-quart enameled cast-iron one that does the trick. Pour the water over the bulgur and cover. Let it steam for about 40 minutes, or until tender.

In the meantime, prepare the rest of the kibbeh.

Preheat a large skillet over medium heat. Sauté the onion in the olive oil for about 5 minutes, until translucent. Add the garlic and sauté for a minute more. Mix in the eggplant, salt, and pepper, cover the pan, and cook for about 15 minutes, stirring occasionally. The eggplant should release a bunch of moisture and cook down.

Preheat the oven to 350°F.

Add the tomatoes and cumin to the skillet and cook for another 10 minutes. Turn off the heat. The bulgur should be done at this point, so add it to the pan and thoroughly combine. Fold in the chopped mint.

Spray an 8-inch square baking pan with nonstick cooking spray. Press the kibbeh firmly into the baking pan. Bake for 25 minutes. It tastes great served warm, but I actually like it even better at room temp, once the flavors have melded. Serve garnished with mint.

ঙ INGREDIENT SCAVENGER HUNT

Bulgur is a toasty cracked wheat that's been parboiled so you can cook it as you would cook couscous, by just steaming it. Unlike couscous, it's a whole grain that's been minimally processed. It's usually found in bulk bins or at a Mediterranean supermarket, but even though it is cracked wheat, it is always labeled "bulgur." If something is simply labeled "cracked wheat," that means it has not been parboiled and the cooking time will be much longer. ঙ

Tamarind Quinoa

SERVES 4 • ACTIVE TIME: 15 MINUTES • TOTAL TIME: 45 MINUTES

PER SERVING
(¼ RECIPE):
Calories: 250
Calories from fat: 50
Total fat: 6 g
Saturated fat: 2 g
Trans fat: 0 g
Total carb: 40 g
Fiber: 5 g
Sugars: 7 g
Protein: 9 g
Cholesterol: 0 mg
Sodium: 490 mg
Vitamin A: 6%
Vitamin C: 8%
Calcium: 6%
Iron: 15%

Looking for a new and fun way to dress up your quinoa? Here's a spin on Indian-inspired tamarind rice that will get your taste buds a-movin'. Serve with any of the curries.

- 1 teaspoon vegetable oil
- ¼ cup minced onion
- 1 tablespoon minced fresh ginger
- 3 cloves garlic, minced
- 2 teaspoons coriander seeds, crushed
- 1 cup quinoa
- 2 cups vegetable broth
- ¼ teaspoon salt
- ½ cup low-fat coconut milk
- 1½ teaspoons tamarind concentrate
- ¼ cup raisins
- ⅓ cup frozen peas
- ¼ cup chopped fresh cilantro

Preheat a 2-quart pot over medium heat. Sauté the onion, ginger, garlic, and coriander seeds in the oil for about 5 minutes, until the onions are translucent. Use a little cooking spray if needed.

Add the quinoa, broth, and salt. Cover and bring to a boil. Once boiling, lower the heat to a simmer and cook, covered, for about 20 minutes, or until most of the water is absorbed, stirring often. The quinoa should be tender and fluffy. Add the coconut milk and tamarind, and stir until the tamarind is completely dissolved. Fold in the raisins, peas, and cilantro. Turn off the heat, but keep covered to warm the peas through—about 5 minutes. Fold in the cilantro and serve.

CHAPTER 3

Rub-Your-Tummy Veggies

VEGETABLES. THIS IS WHAT IT'S ALL ABOUT! THESE ARE WHAT most Americans are seriously lacking in their diet. Nutrients, vitamins, fiber—vegetables have got it all. And, yes, they've got taste, too! Lots of books have been written about sneaking veggies into your diet, and that is, frankly, pathetic. It's like hiding a beautiful princess away in a castle. That glorious asparagus should not have to be boiled to death, pureed, and then stuck into a peanut butter sandwich, or whatever those books are doing to vegetables nowadays. There is no sneaking around here, no smoke and mirrors. We're going to cook veggies, in all their recognizable glory, and by golly, we are going to enjoy them!

While there are a ton of veggies in all the other chapters as well, the recipes in this chapter are really about simple preparation techniques for veggies front and center. It's about using various methods to coax the most flavor out of the vegetable. So you can think about this as a chapter of side dishes, but really what you're getting is a mini-cooking lesson. Broiling, sautéing, roasting, it's all here. And it's time for you to get it all in there (I'm pointing to your belly).

DON'T FEAR THE STEAMER

What's up with steamophobia? For years I suffered from an irrational fear of cooking with steam. I guess it seemed like such a chore: setting up your apparatus, boiling water, peeling, chopping, and all just for what in the end was a pile of vegetables.

Now I know better. I found a steamer that doesn't feel like a hassle, I've got broccoli-chopping down to a science and I have an intense appreciation for that "pile of vegetables." Steaming doesn't have to mean boring! It can be the perfect way to coax the pure and simple flavors out of your produce. Here are a few tips and tricks to help you steam like you mean it.

1. No fancy equipment required. The steamer that I absolutely love is the basket that fits into my 6-quart soup pot. It's big enough so that I don't have to crowd everything in there and it's easy to use—no hard-to-clean sliding parts or things that can fall apart or malfunction. It's also convenient—because I always have my pot resting on the stove, it's not like I have to go shuffling through pots and pans to get to it. The only thing that could be easier is if the veggies would jump into the pot and steam themselves (I'm working on that part).

2. Practice, practice, practice; timing is everything; and other clichés. The more veggies you chop, the quicker it will get. Try steaming veggies at least three days a week and see if you're not Iron Chef material by the end of the month. For best results, prep veggies evenly sized and experiment with different cooking times. Soon you'll know exactly how you like your veggies. Another option is to be a lazyhead and steam things that need minimal prep, such as green beans, baby carrots, and asparagus.

3. Salt! You want to gobble down veggies the same way you eat French fries? A little salt goes a long, long way. And if you take one thing away from this steaming treatise, let it be this: salt before you steam! This way, the salt melts into the veggies, extending the flavor and really sinking in. A few granules at the end of steaming won't have the same effect, and I don't know about you, but soy sauce on steamed veggies tastes a little tedious to me. It covers up the natural, bright flavors. Salt brings those flavors out. Just sprinkle a bit of salt over the veggies right when you add them to the steamer basket and see it light up your life.

4. Herbs! Fresh herbs scattered over your veggies at the onset of cooking really brightens them up. Depending on what you are serving them with, try fresh cilantro, basil, thyme, dill, oregano, or mint. Can you use dried herbs? Yes! But your results may vary. I especially like to use dried oregano.

5. Don't overcook them. If you're mixing several types of veggies, use the **steaming times on the next page** to know which veggies to start with, adding the ones with shorter cooking times as you go along.

6. Don't overpack them. You can get a lot more than a single layer into a steamer basket, but try not to fill it more than three-quarters full, for the most even cooking. If you want to make a lot more veggies, just do two separate batches.

A GUIDE TO A STEAMY LOVE AFFAIR
Use this guide to get your steaming started. In reality, any of the veggies can go with any of the dressings and sauces, but I've given you a few of my favorites. Also, check out the bowl section (page 265) to work steamed veggies into larger meals. I'm giving you basic cooking times, but remember that everyone's equip-

ment and preferences are different, so start here but figure out what works best for you.

Asparagus

Remove the coarse ends. Different-size asparagus call for different cooking times. Steam pencil-thin spears for about 4 minutes, and the fattest spears for 8 minutes. Most asparagus are somewhere in between, so 6 minutes should about do it. The asparagus should turn a pretty Kermit green.
Especially yummy with: **Sanctuary Dressing** (page 29).

Broccoli

Peel the stalk if it seems especially thick. Cut the stalk into ½-inch-thick pieces. Slice the broccoli branches into large florets. Steam the stalks alone for 2 minutes, then add the florets and steam for about 5 more minutes. The broccoli should turn a dark but bright Godzilla green.
Lip-smacking good with: **Orange–Sesame Vinaigrette** (page 43).

Brussels Sprouts

Slice off the little nubby bottom. Slice the larger Brussels sprouts in half and keep the smaller ones whole. Steam for 8 minutes. The leaves should be a glossy lime green.
Comforty good with: **Easy Breezy Cheezy Sauce** (page 173).

Carrots

Use baby carrots for lazy nights. For big carrots, peel and slice them ½ inch thick (on a diagonal, for maximum prettiness). Steam for about 10 minutes.

Simply delectable with: **Roasted Red Pepper & Kalamata Hummus** (page 138).

Cauliflower

Aim for florets that are Ping-Pong ball size. Discard the stems. Steam for about 5 minutes.
Sensuously delicious with: **Caesar Chavez Dressing** (page 43).

Green Beans

Snip off the stems and ends and discard. Steam the beans for no more than 4 minutes. Green beans should turn a brilliant spring green.
Gingery good with: **Carrot Ginger Dressing** (page 52).

Kale

Remove the coarse stems and tear the kale into bite-size pieces. You'll need to flip the kale every few minutes with tongs, so stand by. Cook for about 8 minutes.
Totally droolworthy with: **Balsamic Vinaigrette** (page 17).

Zucchini and Yellow Squash

I'm really careful about steaming zukes and summer squash because they can go from zero to inedible mush so quickly! Slice off the stem and cut the squash into ½-inch pieces (again, bias-cut looks pretty). Check for doneness after 5 minutes. Zucchini should be firm and just turning shimmery inside—not mushy.
Springtime superb with: **Red Velvet Mole** (page 134).

Artichokes

This is for those times when you're feeling a little more adventurous, as there's a bit of prep involved, but mark my words, it's worth it. You'll need plenty of lemon slices for this.

Cut off the tops of the artichokes so that they're relatively flat (so cut about an inch off) and rub with lemon slices. You can use kitchen shears to snip the pointy tips off the leaves, but it isn't totally necessary. Open up the leaves a bit to get to the center. Pull out the choke as best you can, then use a spoon to scoop out the stringy center. Rub the leaves all over with lemon slices, then tuck lemon slices into the leaves. Steam the artichokes upside down for about 40 minutes.

Absolutely mouthwatering with: **Green Goddess Garlic Dressing** (page 26).

STEAMING BENEFITS—USE THE STEAM AND KEEP THE GREEN

And if taste wasn't reason enough to get on board, steaming vegetables offers a number of nutritional advantages.

Fewer nutrients lost: When boiling vegetables, the hot water pulls out water-soluble vitamins such as C and the B vitamins riboflavin, niacin, and folate. Beneficial phytochemicals and antioxidants may also be lost in boiling. The stuff from broccoli that turns the boiling water green is actually what you want to be eating more of!

More nutrients gained: Some vitamins and minerals are found behind tough cell walls and steaming loosens them up, making them more available to your body than if eaten raw. The beta-carotene in carrots is a great example.

More vegetables eaten: One of the many benefits of vegetables is the fiber they contain. Fiber helps to fill you up, which is great when you are trying to eat less, but sometimes we want to eat more vegetables to get all of their nutrients. Steaming softens the fiber so you can eat more. As shown here, steaming also adds to the taste and texture of vegetables. More is better when it comes to vegetables, even when you are trying to lose weight. When you are filling up on nutrient-dense veggies, you are eating less of the high-calorie stuff.

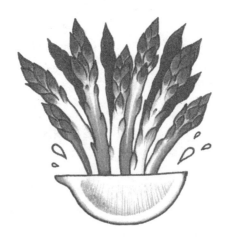

Garlicky Mushrooms & Kale

SERVES 4 • ACTIVE TIME: 10 MINUTES • TOTAL TIME: 20 MINUTES

I probably eat this more than any other recipe in the book, sometimes all on its own, sometimes as a side, sometimes just to impress passersby with how healthy I am. The flavors are so very simple but so satisfying, and they go with most everything. You can use any kind of kale you like: dinosaur, Red Russian, or just plain old dark green Godzilla-lookin' kale. The mushrooms add a meaty bite, and they're also great little containers of flavor, absorbing all that garlicky goodness.

> 1 teaspoon olive oil
> 6 cloves garlic, minced
> ¼ teaspoon salt
> 8 ounces cremini or button mushrooms, sliced (about 2 cups)
> 1 pound kale, coarse stems removed, leaves sliced or torn into pieces
> Several pinches of freshly ground black pepper

Preheat a large skillet over medium heat. Sauté the garlic in the oil for about 2 minutes, being careful not to burn it. Spray it with a little non-stick cooking spray if needed. Add the mushrooms and sprinkle on the

---

PER SERVING
(¼ RECIPE):
Calories: 130
Calories from fat: 30
Total fat: 3 g
Saturated fat: 0 g
Trans fat: 0 g
Total carb: 18 g
Fiber: 5 g
Sugars: 3 g
Protein: 9 g
Cholesterol: 0 mg
Sodium: 380 mg
Vitamin A: 350%
Vitamin C: 230%
Calcium: 15%
Iron: 15%

∾ NUTRITION TIP *There is so much misinformation out there when it comes to calcium. For example, some people believe that calcium is not that important and the big bad dairy industry is just fooling us. Well, the dairy industry may be trying to fool us, but calcium is still important, for more than just bones and teeth. Calcium is an electrolyte, and works in the contraction of muscles (including the heart!) and blood clotting. Fortunately, we have plenty of sources, such as kale. One cup of raw kale has 90 mg, about 10 percent of the daily recommendation, and because it shrinks down so much in cooking, it's easy to eat 4 or 5 cups. ∾*

salt. Let them cook for 5 to 7 minutes, stirring often, until the moisture has released and the mushrooms are lightly browned.

Add the kale and pepper, and use tongs to sauté for about 10 more minutes. Add splashes of water if the pan seems dry. The kale should be tender and cooked down pretty well. Serve immediately.

TIP *Depending on what you're serving this with, you can really cater the flavors to your desires. Add some minced ginger when serving with other gingery dishes, or add a big pinch of thyme if serving with Italian or Thanksgiving-type dishes. If you like it spicy, a big pinch of red pepper flakes is in order.*

Jerk Asparagus

SERVES 4 • ACTIVE TIME: 5 MINUTES • TOTAL TIME: 15 MINUTES

sparagus is kind of fun to chew, so it's a great candidate for jerk spices. Use a cast-iron pan to get the most charred flavor out of your sautéed veggies. I love how the spices in jerk seasoning seem like they won't work together, and then they totally do and you feel like a jerk for thinking otherwise. Unfortunately, that's not where the name came from. Serve over rice, alongside **Caribbean Curried Black-Eyed Peas with Plantains** (page 129), or with **Mango BBQ Beans** (page 133) .

1 teaspoon olive oil
2 teaspoons minced fresh ginger
4 cloves garlic, minced
¼ teaspoon red pepper flakes (or more if you like it spicy)
¼ teaspoon dried thyme
1 pound asparagus, coarse ends removed
¼ teaspoon salt
¼ teaspoon allspice
Pinch of ground nutmeg
Pinch of ground cinnamon
Lime wedges, to serve

PER SERVING
(¼ RECIPE):
Calories: 40
Calories from fat: 10
Total fat: 1.5 g
Saturated fat: 0 g
Trans fat: 0 g
Total carb: 6 g
Fiber: 2 g
Sugars: 2 g
Protein: 3 g
Cholesterol: 0 mg
Sodium: 150 mg
Vitamin A: 15%
Vitamin C: 10%
Calcium: 4%
Iron: 15%

Preheat a large, heavy-bottomed skillet over medium-high heat. Sauté the ginger and garlic in the oil for about 30 seconds. Add the red pepper flakes and thyme, plus a splash of water. Let it sizzle for a few seconds. Add the asparagus, salt, and spices. Use tongs to toss and coat, adding a few splashes of water if it seems dry. Sauté for about 10 minutes, until the asparagus is tender and the ends are slightly frizzled. Serve immediately.

∾ TIP *For sautéed recipes, I generally prefer to use asparagus that's on the thin side and save those fat stalks for the grill or broiler.* ∾

Shaved Brussels Sprouts

SERVES 4 • ACTIVE TIME: 20 MINUTES • TOTAL TIME: 25 MINUTES

PER SERVING
(¼ RECIPE):
Calories: 70
Calories from fat: 15
Total fat: 1.5 g
Saturated fat: 0 g
Trans fat: 0 g
Total carb: 12 g
Fiber: 5 g
Sugars: 3 g
Protein: 4 g
Cholesterol: 0 mg
Sodium: 170 mg
Vitamin A: 15%
Vitamin C: 160%
Calcium: 6%
Iron: 10%

When you thinly slice Brussels sprouts and cook them over high heat, they take on a whole new dimension. The outer layer gets toasty and crispy, the inner leaves remain intact and stay firm and crunchy. I like to use them as a garnish as well as a side, so sprinkle them over BBQ dishes or drop 'em on savory gravy entrées. They'll add a fun flavor and texture.

  1   teaspoon olive oil
  ¼   cup thinly sliced onion
  6   cloves garlic, sliced thinly
  1   pound thinly sliced Brussels sprouts (see tip)
  ¼   teaspoon salt
       Freshly ground black pepper

Preheat a large, heavy skillet over medium-high heat. Cast iron works best here to get the sprouts nice and crispy. Sauté the onion in oil for about 3 minutes, until just starting to brown. Add the garlic and sauté for another 30 seconds. Add the Brussels sprouts, salt, and pepper. Sauté for about 7 minutes, until the leaves are browned and crisped. They're ready!

> **TIP** To get the Brussels sprouts "shaved," no need to break out the straight-edge razor. Trim the nub on the bottom and slice the sprout in half lengthwise. Then just slice the sprouts into thin-as-you-can lengthwise strips. It might take a bit of time, but it's a great way to enjoy these little guys and well worth it!

Pineapple Collards

SERVES 4 • ACTIVE TIME: 10 MINUTES • TOTAL TIME: 20 MINUTES

I was in a greens rut. I wanted something sour and tangy for my greens but I'd been putting lime in *everything* and needed a change. Pineapple totally worked! It's a fun twist with just a hint of juicy sweetness. These are perfect served with **Broiled Blackened Tofu** (page 147) and **Butternut Coconut Rice** (page 80), or for any dinner when you need to get out of your greens rut.

- 1 teaspoon sesame oil
- 6 cloves garlic, minced
- 2 teaspoons minced fresh ginger
- ¼ teaspoon red pepper flakes
- 1 pound collards, coarse stems removed, leaves torn into bite-size pieces
- ½ cup pineapple, chopped finely
- ¼ teaspoon salt

PER SERVING
(¼ RECIPE):
Calories: 60
Calories from fat: 15
Total fat: 1.5 g
Saturated fat: 0 g
Trans fat: 0 g
Total carb: 11 g
Fiber: 4 g
Sugars: 2 g
Protein: 3 g
Cholesterol: 0 mg
Sodium: 170 mg
Vitamin A: 150%
Vitamin C: 80%
Calcium: 20%
Iron: 8%

Preheat a large skillet over medium heat. Sauté the garlic, ginger, and red pepper flakes in the oil for about 2 minutes, being careful not to burn them. Spray them with a little nonstick cooking spray if needed. Add the collards, pineapple, and salt, and use tongs to sauté for about 10 more minutes. Use splashes of water if the pan seems dry. The collards should be tender and cooked down pretty well. Serve immediately.

> ❧ TIP I prefer to use fresh pineapple, but canned will work if you use the kind packed in only juice (not syrup). ❧

Creamed Corn

SERVES 4 • ACTIVE TIME: 15 MINUTES • TOTAL TIME: 25 MINUTES

~~~~~~~~~~~~~~~
PER SERVING
(¼ RECIPE):
Calories: 130
Calories from fat: 30
Total fat: 3.5 g
Saturated fat: 0 g
Trans fat: 0 g
Total carb: 23 g
Fiber: 4 g
Sugars: 4 g
Protein: 5 g
Cholesterol: 0 mg
Sodium: 310 mg
Vitamin A: 0%
Vitamin C: 10%
Calcium: 0%
Iron: 6%

Creamed corn is such a heavenly backdrop for so many things. Latin dishes, Southern dishes, barbecue; I keep the flavor simple so it can go with almost anything. Sautéing the corn before blending it gives it an added depth of flavor. Although this is best with fresh corn, if using frozen allow for 5 more minutes cooking time when you sauté the corn.

½ cup plus ⅓ cup plain unsweetened almond milk
1 tablespoon cornstarch
1 teaspoon olive oil
3 cups fresh corn (from about 3 ears)
½ teaspoon salt

Mix ⅓ cup of the almond milk with the cornstarch and set aside.

Preheat a 4-quart heavy-bottomed pan over medium-high heat. Sauté the corn in the vegetable oil for about 5 minutes, until tender, with flecks of brown in places. Sprinkle with the salt.

Add the ½ cup almond milk (not the ⅓ cup with the cornstarch) and blend with an immersion blender until about two-thirds of the corn is pureed and there are still some whole or half pieces left. If you don't have an immersion blender, then transfer the mixture to a blender and pulse to the desired consistency, then transfer back to the pot. Turn up the heat to medium.

Add the cornstarch mixture and stir constantly until thickened, 5 to 7 minutes. Serve immediately.

> ∾ **NUTRITION TIP** *You are the salt of the earth! Sodium is a required nutrient and naturally occurs in such vegetables as corn. It is an electrolyte that maintains our fluid balance and is essential for our muscles. Careful, though. Too much salt and sodium are associated with high blood pressure and hypertension. Try to stay cool and collected and keep your daily salt intake at 2,300 mg per day.* ∾

Mushroom Tibs

SERVES 4 • ACTIVE TIME: 15 MINUTES • TOTAL TIME: 40 MINUTES

One of my favorite restaurants in Portland is called E'njoni. They call themselves "Eritrean Mediterranean," and although you will find many of the familiar Ethiopian restaurant staples, the pureed veggies and stews, what I love about it there is that you'll also find dishes like this—mushroom tibs: spicy and oh-so-flavorful mushrooms with curry, warm cloves, and floral thyme. Serve with **Ethiopian Millet** (page 78) and **Ye'abesha Gomen** (page 109).

- 1 pound cremini mushrooms, sliced in half
- 1 teaspoon oil
- 1 tablespoon tomato paste
- ⅓ cup vegetable broth
- 3 cloves garlic, minced
- 2 teaspoons minced fresh ginger
- ¼ teaspoon cayenne
- 2 teaspoons mild curry powder
- 1 teaspoon Hungarian paprika
- 2 teaspoons ground cumin
- 2 teaspoons dried thyme
- ¼ teaspoon ground cardamom
- ⅛ teaspoon ground cloves
- ½ teaspoon salt

PER SERVING
(¼ RECIPE):
Calories: 50
Calories from fat: 5
Total fat: 0.5 g
Saturated fat: 0 g
Trans fat: 0 g
Total carb: 9 g
Fiber: 2 g
Sugars: 3 g
Protein: 4 g
Cholesterol: 0 mg
Sodium: 350 mg
Vitamin A: 8%
Vitamin C: 4%
Calcium: 6%
Iron: 10%

> **NUTRITION TIP** *Poor mushrooms are so misunderstood. They get a bad rap as "mostly water," but the truth is they are a very good source of copper, riboflavin, niacin, and selenium. Copper works with iron and is vital in the formation of hemoglobin—the stuff in your blood that keeps your oxygen flowing. And what's more, a cup of mushrooms has only 20 measly calories.*

Preheat the oven to 400°F.

Place the mushrooms in an 8 by 13-inch metal baking pan. In a cup, use a fork to mix together the oil, tomato paste, and vegetable broth. Add the remainder of the ingredients and mix well.

Coat the mushrooms with the mixture. Bake for 15 minutes, remove from the oven, and toss. Add a little vegetable broth if it appears too dry. Return to the oven and bake for 5 more minutes. The mushrooms should be coated with a thick paste of spice; if it seems too thick, thin it out with a bit of vegetable broth or water. Taste for salt and serve.

TIP *If you're a spice wuss, then omit the cayenne. You'll still have some spiciness from the curry.*

Braised Cabbage with Seitan

SERVES 4 • ACTIVE TIME: 20 MINUTES • TOTAL TIME: 30 MINUTES

This ain't your grandma's cabbage! Actually, was your grandma really good at making cabbage? Then this *might* be hers. Don't be fooled by the short ingredient list; braising is the best thing you can do for your cabbage. It makes it tender and flavorful without becoming mushy, and the simmered broth tastes great over potatoes or rice. The seitan adds flavor, protein, and a chewy texture that might make this more of a main than a side. Serve with a baked potato, sweet or regular, or some basmati rice.

1 teaspoon olive oil
1½ cups seitan, sliced ¼ inch thick
4 cloves garlic, minced
2 teaspoons dried thyme
¼ teaspoon red pepper flakes
2 cups vegetable broth
1 pound green cabbage, cut into thin strips (about 4 cups)
¼ teaspoon salt

PER SERVING
(¼ RECIPE):
Calories: 150
Calories from fat: 30
Total fat: 3.5 g
Saturated fat: 0 g
Trans fat: 0 g
Total carb: 14 g
Fiber: 3 g
Sugars: 5 g
Protein: 18 g
Cholesterol: 0 mg
Sodium: 590
Vitamin A: 2%
Vitamin C: 70%
Calcium: 10%
Iron: 10%

Preheat a large skillet over medium heat. Sauté the seitan in oil until lightly browned, about 7 minutes. Use nonstick cooking spray as needed. Add the garlic, thyme, and red pepper flakes, and sauté for a minute more. Add a splash of the vegetable broth to deglaze the pan, then add the cabbage and the rest of the broth. Sprinkle with salt. Cover the pan and cook for 15 minutes, stirring occasionally. The cabbage should be tender with just a little bit of snap to it. Taste for salt and serve immediately.

Green Beans with Thai Basil

SERVES 4 • ACTIVE TIME: 15 MINUTES • TOTAL TIME: 30 MINUTES

(CAN BE MADE GLUTEN FREE IF USING GF TAMARI IN PLACE OF SOY SAUCE)

If you like your springtime a little spicy, this side dish is for you! Green beans are coated in a slightly sweet soy sauce, punctuated with shallot, ginger, and garlic. Fragrant and sweet Thai basil brings notes of licorice that will transport you, if not to Thailand, then at least a little beyond Thai take-out. Serve with **Bhutanese Pineapple Rice** (page 72) and **Red Thai Tofu** (page 149).

1	teaspoon olive oil
¼	cup thinly sliced shallot
2	teaspoon minced fresh ginger
3	cloves garlic, minced
1	pound green beans, ends removed
¼	teaspoon red pepper flakes
1	tablespoon soy sauce
1	tablespoon agave nectar
2	tablespoons freshly squeezed lime juice
	About 15 leaves fresh Thai basil

∾ INGREDIENT SCAVENGER HUNT

Thai basil isn't the easiest herb to find if you don't live near a Chinatown or an Asian market. Such places as Whole Foods Market often have it, though, and many greengrocers and farmers' markets will keep it in stock when it's in season. I would highly recommend growing your own, because the flavor is so special and tasty that you really shouldn't live your life without it. ∾

Preheat a large skillet over medium high heat. Sauté the shallot in oil for about 5 minutes, or until translucent. Add the garlic and ginger and sauté for about 30 seconds more. Add the green beans and cook for about 5 minutes, stirring often. Add the red pepper flakes, soy sauce, agave, and lime juice. Cook for around 5 more minutes, stirring often. The green beans should still have some crunch. Stir in the basil, turn off the heat, and let the basil wilt. Serve!

> ∾ TIP *Want to turn this into a main dish? Dry-fry a block of tofu, then add it back to the dish near the end of the cooking time, for about 5 minutes.* ∾

Orange-Scented Broccoli

SERVES 4 • ACTIVE TIME: 10 MINUTES • TOTAL TIME: 20 MINUTES

(CAN BE MADE GLUTEN FREE IF USING GF TAMARI IN PLACE OF SOY SAUCE)

~~~~~~~~~~~~~
PER SERVING
(¼ RECIPE):
Calories: 80
Calories from fat: 15
Total fat: 1.5 g
Saturated fat: 0 g
Trans fat: 0 g
Total carb: 14 g
Fiber: 4 g
Sugars: 5 g
Protein: 4 g
Cholesterol: 0 mg
Sodium: 330 mg
Vitamin A: 20%
Vitamin C: 230%
Calcium: 8%
Iron: 6%

A fun way to liven up broccoli when you're tired of the same-old same-old. This broccoli goes great with Asian-themed meals. Mirin isn't totally essential, but it gives the broccoli a fragrant and sweet flavor. You can sub a little white wine if you must, though.

- 1 teaspoon sesame oil
- 1 tablespoon minced fresh ginger
- 3 cloves garlic
- ½ teaspoon red pepper flakes
- 1 bunch broccoli (about 1¼ pounds), stems thinly sliced, tops cut into florets
- 1 tablespoon mirin
- 1 tablespoon soy sauce
- 2 teaspoons orange zest
- ¼ cup freshly squeezed orange juice

Preheat a large skillet over medium heat. Sauté the ginger in the oil for about 2 minutes. Add the garlic and red pepper flakes and sauté for a minute more. Use nonstick cooking spray or a splash of water if things are sticking.

Add the broccoli, mirin, and soy sauce. Sauté for around 7 more minutes, tossing frequently, until the stalks are tender. Add the zest and orange juice, and sauté for a minute more. Serve immediately.

∾ NUTRITION TIP

We don't exactly associate broccoli with protein, but would you believe that more than 25 percent of the calories in broccoli are from protein? Well, believe it! 'Cause it's true! ∾

Eggplant Dengaku

SERVES 4 • ACTIVE TIME: 20 MINUTES • TOTAL TIME: 30 MINUTES

(CAN BE MADE GLUTEN FREE IF USING GF TAMARI IN PLACE OF SOY SAUCE)

 staple on Japanese restaurant menus, this eggplant is broiled and coasted in a rich, pungent, and slightly sweet miso sauce. I'm not usually a stickler for a particular type of miso, but here I insist that you use red miso for the most authentic taste. And by authentic I mean Japanese-American restaurant authentic, because I'm just a nice Jewish girl who has never actually been to Japan. Serve this over brown rice or alongside the **Sushi Roll Edamame Salad** (page 20) or the **Miso Udon Stir-fry with Greens and Beans** (page 182).

- ¼ cup mirin
- 2 teaspoons soy sauce
- 2 tablespoons water
- 5 teaspoons agave
- ¼ cup red miso
- 2 pounds eggplant, cut ½ inch thick
  Sliced scallions, for garnish (optional)

PER SERVING
(¼ RECIPE):
Calories: 130
Calories from fat: 15
Total fat: 1.5 g
Saturated fat: 0 g
Trans fat: 0 g
Total carb: 28 g
Fiber: 10 g
Sugars: 11 g
Protein: 3 g
Cholesterol: 0 mg
Sodium: 930 mg
Vitamin A: 0%
Vitamin C: 8%
Calcium: 6%
Iron: 4%

In a saucepot, combine the mirin, soy sauce and agave. Bring to a boil and then lower the heat. Add the agave and miso. Stir over very low heat, whisking often, until it is smooth.

Preheat the broiler and place a rack about 6 inches from the heat. Spray a large rimmed baking sheet with nonstick cooking spray. Arrange the eggplant slices in a single layer and spray lightly with cooking spray. Broil for about 6 minutes; the tops should be browned and the eggplant should be cooked but still a bit firm. Remove from the oven.

Use a tablespoon to divide the miso sauce among all the eggplant slices, then use the back of the spoon to spread on each entire slice. Place back in the broiler and broil for 2 more minutes. The miso should be a little bubbly. Serve as soon as you can.

> ✑ NOTE *1 teaspoon of oil has been added to the nutritional info to allow for the nonstick cooking spray.* ✑

Coriander Mushrooms with Cherry Tomatoes

SERVES 4 • ACTIVE TIME: 15 MINUTES • TOTAL TIME: 20 MINUTES

These mushrooms pop with some of my favorite flavors in the world: aromatic coriander, fruity jalapeños, earthy mushrooms, and piquant tomatoes. I find them irresistible alongside **Unfried Refried Beans** (page 136) or tucked into tacos on taco night.

1 teaspoon olive oil
4 cloves garlic, minced
2 jalapeños, seeded and sliced thinly
1 tablespoon coriander seeds, crushed (see tip page 102)
1 pound cremini mushrooms, sliced
1 cup cherry tomatoes, sliced in half
2 teaspoons dried oregano
  Several pinches of freshly ground black pepper
¼ teaspoon salt
1 tablespoon freshly squeezed lime juice
  Fresh cilantro, for garnish (optional)

Preheat a large skillet over medium-low heat. Sauté the the garlic, jalapeños, and coriander seeds in oil for about 5 minutes, to soften the seeds. Stir frequently to avoid burning the garlic; add splashes of water if things start sticking. Turn up the heat to medium; add the mushrooms, tomatoes, oregano, salt, and black pepper, and sauté for about 10 minutes, until the mushrooms are softened and the tomatoes are cooked down. Taste for salt and serve garnished with fresh cilantro, if you like.

Grilled Portobellos

SERVES 4 • ACTIVE TIME: 15 MINUTES • TOTAL TIME: 20 MINUTES

(CAN BE MADE GLUTEN FREE IF USING GF TAMARI IN PLACE OF SOY SAUCE)

Juicy, sloppy, meaty portobellos. This is what you want to serve over pasta, in a burger, over a salad, or just alongside mashed potatoes and gravy. Master the art of the portobello and you've opened up a world of culinary bliss that will last you a lifetime of dinners. The versatile flavors of the basic marinade go with almost anything, but try some of the variations, too.

4 portobello caps, stems removed

MARINADE:

½ cup dry white wine

2 teaspoons olive oil

2 tablespoons balsamic vinegar

2 tablespoons tamari or soy sauce

2 cloves garlic, minced

1 teaspoon liquid smoke

PER SERVING
(1 PORTOBELLO CAP):
Calories: 80
Calories from fat: 20
Total fat: 2.5 g
Saturated fat: 0 g
Trans fat: 0 g
Total carb: 8 g
Fiber: 3 g
Sugars: 3 g
Protein: 4 g
Cholesterol: 0 mg
Sodium: 700 mg
Vitamin A: 0%
Vitamin C: 0%
Calcium: 4%
Iron: 4%

Place the portobellos gills up in a rimmed baking sheet. Mix all the marinade ingredients together and spoon over the portobellos. Let marinate for at least half an hour, sporking the marinade back onto the mushrooms every 10 minutes or so.

Preheat your grill over medium high. Spray it with nonstick cooking spray. Place the portobellos gills up on the grill, and cover. Cook for about 5 minutes; there should be grill marks on the caps. Flip over, cover, and cook for about 3 more minutes. Your cooking time may vary depending on the size of your portobellos and the temperature of your grill. You know the mushrooms are done when you press on the center (where the stem used to be) with tongs and it's very soft and juicy. To serve, let them sit on the cutting board for a few minutes to cool off for a bit, then slice into ½-inch pieces. I like them best when sliced at an angle. Serve warm!

Variations

Masala Portobellos: Use the **Masala Baked Tofu Marinade** (page 146).
Portobello Chimichurri: Use the **Tofu Chimichurri Marinade** (page 150).
BBQ Portos: Use the **Tamarind BBQ Sauce** (page 159).
Buffabellos: Use the **Buffalo Tempeh Marinade** (page 161).

TIP *Don't have a cast-iron grill? Don't worry! A broiler is the next best thing. Follow the directions, but instead of grilling, broil for about 5 minutes on each side.*

Sweet & Salty Maple Baby Carrots

SERVES 4 • ACTIVE TIME: 3 MINUTES • TOTAL TIME: 40 MINUTES

A few simple ingredients transform baby carrots into sublime morsels that you can't help but pop into your mouth. These are the perfect accompaniment to an autumn comfort food meal, such as mashed **Caulipots** (page 54) and **Silky Chickpea Gravy** (page 56).

- 1 pound baby carrots
- 2 tablespoons pure maple syrup
- ½ teaspoon kosher salt

Preheat the oven to 375°F.

Line an 8-inch square baking dish with tinfoil and spray with cooking spray. Put the carrots in the pan and drizzle with the syrup. Sprinkle with the salt and toss to coat. Cover with foil and bake for 30 minutes. Remove from the oven, flip the carrots, and bake for another 10 minutes, uncovered. Serve immediately.

PER SERVING
(¼ RECIPE):
Calories: 70
Calories from fat: 0
Total fat: 0 g
Saturated fat: 0 g
Trans fat: 0 g
Total carb: 16 g
Fiber: 3 g
Sugars: 11 g
Protein: <1 g
Cholesterol: 0 mg
Sodium: 330 mg
Vitamin A: 310%
Vitamin C: 4%
Calcium: 4%
Iron: 6%

> **NUTRITION TIP** Cooking carrots breaks down their tough fibrous walls and increases the availability of some nutrients. Carrots are known for beta-carotene, which is both a precursor to vitamin A and an antioxidant, but also contain a phytochemical called falcarinol that may protect against cancer.

Five-Spice Delicata Squash

SERVES 4 • ACTIVE TIME: 10 MINUTES • TOTAL TIME: 50 MINUTES

Delicata is the golden child of squash; it's tender, sweet, creamy, and best of all, you don't have to peel it; you can eat the skin. I've been using this water bath/tinfoil method to cook delicata for as long as I can remember . . . way before the Internet told us how to cook things. I think it brings out the most flavor without adding a ton of (vegan) butter. Five-spice is a perfect blend for squash: star anise, cinnamon, and, uh, three other spices, I suppose. It just brings out the best.

- 2 average-size delicata squash, sliced in half lenghwise, seeds removed
- 4 teaspoons pure maple syrup
- 1 teaspoon Chinese five-spice powder
- 1 teaspoon salt

Preheat the oven to 425°F. Fill an 8 by 13-inch baking pan with about 1½ inches of water. Place the squashes in the water, cut side up. Drizzle each slice with a teaspoon of maple syrup, then sprinkle evenly with the five-spice and salt. Wrap with tinfoil and bake for about 45 minutes, or until the squash is pierced easily with a fork. Serve warm.

Sautéed Escarole

SERVES 4 • ACTIVE TIME: 10 MINUTES • TOTAL TIME: 20 MINUTES

I f I see escarole on the menu at an Italian restaurant, I have no choice. I am compelled to order it! So if you've got an Italian menu planned, it must include escarole. It's divine served with **Chickpea Piccata** (page 115) and **Caulipots** (page 54), or with **Basic Baked Tofu** (page 144).

If you've never had escarole before, it looks more like lettuce than do the dark leafy greens you may be used to cooking with. So don't be confused and leave the store in a huff! Escarole sautés just perfectly; the tops of the leaves get mellow and wilted, while closer to the bottom they remain crisp and toothsome. An excellent texture combination.

1 teaspoon olive oil
6 cloves garlic, sliced thinly
1 pound escarole, cored and chopped coarsely
1 teaspoon dried thyme
¼ teaspoon red pepper flakes
Freshly ground black pepper
⅓ cup capers with some brine
Salt
Lemon wedges, for serving

PER SERVING
(¼ RECIPE):
Calories: 40
Calories from fat: 15
Total fat: 1.5 g
Saturated fat: 0 g
Trans fat: 0 g
Total carb: 6 g
Fiber: 4 g
Sugars: 0 g
Protein: 2 g
Cholesterol: 0 mg
Sodium: 360 mg
Vitamin A: 50%
Vitamin C: 15%
Calcium: 8%
Iron: 6%

Preheat a large skillet over medium heat. Sauté the garlic in the olive oil for about 3 minutes, until just starting to brown. Add the escarole along with the thyme, red pepper flakes, black pepper, and a pinch of salt, using tongs to toss until it begins to wilt and release moisture. Add the capers and cook just until heated through, about 3 more minutes. Taste for salt and serve with the lemon wedges.

Herb-Roasted Cauliflower & Bread Crumbs

SERVES 4 • ACTIVE TIME: 10 MINUTES • TOTAL TIME: 25 MINUTES

A light layer of bread crumbs with fragrant herbs will have you popping this cauliflower into your mouth as if it's popcorn. I love this cauliflower to top off spaghetti, alongside lasagne, or tossed into a salad.

⅓ cup store-bought whole wheat bread crumbs
2 teaspoons dried thyme
1 teaspoon dried oregano
1 teaspoon dried basil
½ teaspoon salt
Several pinches of freshly ground black pepper
1 pound cauliflower, cored and chopped into bite-size pieces

Preheat the oven to 425°F. Line a large, rimmed baking sheet with parchment paper and spray with nonstick cooking spray. Set aside.

In a mixing bowl, mix together the bread crumbs, herbs, salt, and pepper. Drizzle in the oil and use your fingertips to rub it into the bread crumbs.

The cauliflower should be slightly damp from having washed it; if it's totally dry then run it under water for a sec, so that the crumbs stick better. Roll the cauliflower around in the crumbs, then place the cauliflower in a single layer on a baking sheet. Sprinkle any excess crumbs over the cauliflower. Spray with a bit of cooking spray.

Bake for 12 minutes, until tender and lightly browned.

Ye'abesha Gomen
(Stewed & Sautéed Collards)

SERVES 4 • ACTIVE TIME: 20 MINUTES • TOTAL TIME: 40 MINUTES

I don't usually cook the living daylights out of my greens, but collards are brought to new heights when they are cooked so tender and off the stem. Ethiopian restaurants serve these mellow stewed and sautéed greens alongside heavily seasoned items, and you should do the same. Try the **Mushroom Tibs** (page 95) and **Ethiopian Millet** (page 78).

PER SERVING
(¼ RECIPE):
Calories: 90
Calories from fat: 15
Total fat: 2 g
Saturated fat: 0 g
Trans fat: 0 g
Total carb: 14 g
Fiber: 7 g
Sugars: 3 g
Protein: 6 g
Cholesterol: 0 mg
Sodium: 310 mg
Vitamin A: 230%
Vitamin C: 100%
Calcium: 25%
Iron: 4%

- 1½ pounds collard greens, coarse stems removed, leaves torn into pieces
- 2 cups vegetable broth
- 1 teaspoon olive oil
- 1 small onion, chopped finely
- 3 cloves garlic, minced
- 1 tablespoon minced fresh ginger
- ½ teaspoon red pepper flakes
- Salt

Place the collards and broth in a 4-quart pot, cover, and bring to a boil. Once boiling, lower the heat to a low boil, and keep covered for about 30 minutes, using tongs to toss the collards around every few minutes. They should become a few shades lighter, and very tender but not complete mush.

When the greens are pretty much ready, preheat a large skillet over medium heat. Sauté the onion, garlic, and ginger in the oil for about 5 minutes, until the onion is translucent. Mix in the red pepper flakes. Use tongs to lift the collards out of the pot and add them to the pan. Don't add the cooking liquid at this point, but do reserve it.

Cook the collards with the onions for about 5 minutes, and add splashes of the reserved broth as needed to keep them from sticking. Taste for salt and serve.

Variations

Feeling collardy but not ginger and peppery? Leave out the pepper flakes and ginger and up the garlic by two cloves. These collards are now ready to go with whatever your little heart desires.

> ❧ NUTRITION TIP *If there were a Calcium Olympics, then greens might take home the gold. Put one serving of these collards against one cup of 2% cow's milk and you'll find that they're almost identical (267 vs. 286 mg), but collards will take the lead in fiber (7 vs. 0 grams) and saturated fat (0 vs. 3 grams). Plus, this dish is lower in overall fat (2 vs. 5 grams) and lower in calories (90 vs. 122).* ❧

Curried Cabbage & Peas

SERVES 4 • ACTIVE TIME: 10 MINUTES • TOTAL TIME: 30 MINUTES

A hearty cabbage side dish, with a little sweet earthiness from carrots and peas. This would be at home alongside any of the Indian-inspired meals, or the Ethiopian dishes. You can try it with plain old brown basmati and **Masala Baked Tofu** (page 146).

- 1 teaspoon olive oil
- 1 small onion, sliced thinly
- 3 cloves garlic, minced
- 1 tablespoon minced fresh ginger
- 1 medium-size carrot, sliced ½ inch thick, diagonally
- 1 pound cabbage, cut into thin strips (about 4 cups, or ½ medium head of cabbage)
- ½ teaspoon salt
- 2 tablespoons curry powder
- ½ to ¾ cup vegetable broth
- 1 cup frozen peas

Preheat a large skillet over medium heat. Sauté the onion in the olive oil with a pinch of salt for about 5 minutes, until translucent. Add the garlic and ginger, and sauté for a minute more. Add a splash of the vegetable broth to deglaze the pan, then add the carrot, cabbage, salt, curry powder, and ½ cup of the vegetable broth. Cover the pan and cook for 10 minutes, stirring occasionally. If needed, add up to ¼ cup more broth.

Add the peas and cook for about 5 minutes. The cabbage should be tender with just a little bit of snap to it. Taste for salt and serve immediately.

PER SERVING
(¼ RECIPE):
Calories: 100
Calories from fat: 15
Total fat: 2 g
Saturated fat: 0 g
Trans fat: 0 g
Total carb: 19 g
Fiber: 6 g
Sugars: 8 g
Protein: 5 g
Cholesterol: 0 mg
Sodium: 430 mg
Vitamin A: 70%
Vitamin C: 90%
Calcium: 8%
Iron: 10%

NUTRITION TIP *This recipe is a great example of the nutrient density of vegetables. In only 100 calories you get 5 grams of protein, 90 milligrams of calcium, and 2 grams of iron—that's no typo, each serving really does have 2 grams of iron. Some is from the cabbage and peas but a surprising source of iron is actually curry powder.*

CHAPTER 4

Main Event Beans

Beans are a staple food in practically every culture, and can the entire world be wrong? Well, maybe, but not about beans! Protein, iron, fiber, calcium—beans are the gift that keep on giving.

And lucky for me that beans are so nutritionally perfect. As a young vegetarian in the '80s, I had to learn new and fun ways to prepare them. Instead of using highly processed and way expensive meat substitutes, I would use beans as my protein. Good thing those fake meats were so expensive, because it gave me a chance to become a connoisseur—to really experience the nuance of each and every bean—taste, texture, and flavor. Every variety has its own unique personality. Rice and beans don't mean deprivation!

Linguistically speaking, *meat* used to mean "beans." And it's not a wholly unfair comparison. Nutritionally speaking, beans are as high in protein as many meats. Beans actually do contain all of the essential amino acids, and if you're eating a variety of plant-based foods, you're set up to have them in the amounts you need. See the bowls section (page 265) to see how it's done! And you know what beans do have that meat does not? Fiber and complex carbohydrates—your body's preferred fuel. Most beans are very low in saturated fat and high in the healthy ones. Plus, the nutrients are so plentiful that it doesn't take many to improve the nutrition of a meal.

This chapter celebrates the endless versatility of beans—lightly mashed, pureed, left whole and stewed, or formed into burgers, beans can be enjoyed every which way. They don't have to be relegated to a side dish. Have your beans front and center as the main event!

Canned vs. Dried: Two Beans Enter, One Bean Leaves

You can't beat canned beans when it comes to convenience and even canned beans are relatively inexpensive. But dried beans *are* cheaper, and there's a certain amount of satisfaction that comes from doing it the old-fashioned way.

To get your beans cooked to perfection, it's best to soak them a day ahead of the big simmer. This softens up the beans and ensures that they cook evenly. Put your dried beans in a pot with plenty of water (water should be 2 or 3 inches above the beans), cover, and stash in the fridge until the next day.

After beans have soaked, drain the water, then replace with fresh, cold water (roughly 3 cups of water to every cup of soaked beans, better too much than too little), and a teaspoon of salt and bring to a boil. Once boiling, lower the heat to a simmer so as not to turn them to mush. Cook with the cover slightly ajar so that steam can escape. How long will depend on the bean but note that different factors, such as how old and how dry the bean is, will affect cooking times. Once the beans are nice and tender, drain and use them as called for in the recipe. One cup of dried beans will yield roughly 3 cups of cooked (results may vary).

Does salt really toughen the beans? Not that I have noticed! Go ahead and add the salt; it really benefits the flavor.

For best results, cook a pound of beans at a time, store in the fridge, and use through-out the week. Some people prefer to freeze beans and have them on hand ad infinitum, and that's fine if you swing that way. I tend to forget items left in my freezer. Below are a few of the beans used throughout this section (and throughout the book) and their approximate cooking times.

Black Beans: 1½ hours
Black-Eyed Peas: 1 hour
Chickpeas (aka Garbanzos): 1½ hours
Great Northern Beans or Navy Beans (White beans): 1½ hours
Kidney Beans or Cannellini Beans: 1 hour
Pinto: 1½ hours

The More You Eat, the More You Toot?

Well, obviously we have to address the musical issues of beans. But there are a few things you can do to minimize the damage! Rinsing canned beans helps, as does changing the soaking liquid when you're cooking dried beans. Another thing that is rumored to help is a seaweed called kombu. It's available in most Asian markets or in large health food stores. Just add a stick of it to your beans while they cook. Kombu also adds a delicious savory and salty flavor.

Chickpea Piccata

SERVES 4 • ACTIVE TIME: 15 MINUTES • TOTAL TIME: 30 MINUTES

A plate of piccata is like an instant fancy dinner with all the stops. One second you're just sitting there, all normal-like, but the moment that first forkful of lemony wine bliss touches your tongue, you're transported to candlelight and tablecloths, even if you're sitting in front of the TV watching *Dancing with the Stars*. This version is made with chickpeas, which make it super fast, and it's served over arugula for some green. I know lots of people are accustomed to piccata with pasta, and that is the Italian tradition, but my first piccata was as a vegan and we vegans love our mashed potatoes, so that is what I suggest serving it with. Try it with the **Caulipots** (page 54).

PER SERVING
(¼ RECIPE):
Calories: 190
Calories from fat: 30
Total fat: 3.5 g
Saturated fat: 0 g
Trans fat: 0 g
Total carb: 30 g
Fiber: 5 g
Sugars: 6 g
Protein: 9 g
Cholesterol: 0 mg
Sodium: 730 mg
Vitamin A: 20%
Vitamin C: 25%
Calcium: 10%
Iron: 15%

1 teaspoon olive oil

1 scant cup thinly sliced shallots

6 cloves garlic, sliced thinly

2 tablespoons bread crumbs

2 cups vegetable broth

⅓ cup dry white wine

A few pinches of freshly ground black pepper

A generous pinch of dried thyme

1 (16-ounce) can chickpeas, drained and rinsed

¼ cup capers with a little brine

3 tablespoons freshly squeezed lemon juice

4 cups arugula

Preheat a large, heavy-bottomed pan over medium heat. Sauté the shallots and garlic for about 5 minutes, until golden. Add the bread crumbs and toast them by stirring constantly for about 2 minutes. They should turn a few shades darker.

Add the vegetable broth, wine, salt, pepper, and thyme. Turn up the heat, bring the mixture to a rolling boil, and let the sauce reduce by half; it should take about 7 minutes.

> **～ TIP**
> *Bulk it up by adding a thinly sliced portobello to the finished dish (try the* **Grilled Portobellos,** *page 103). ～*

Add the chickpeas and capers and let heat through, about 3 minutes. Add the lemon juice and turn off the heat.

If you're serving the piccata with mashed potatoes, place the arugula in a wide bowl. Place the mashed potatoes on top of the arugula and ladle the piccata over the potatoes. The arugula will wilt and it will be lovely. If you are serving the piccata solo, just pour it right over the arugula.

> ∾ TIP Regular old whole wheat bread crumbs work just great in this dish, but try using Italian-flavored ones for even more flavor. ∾

Upside-Down Lentil Shepherd's Pie

SERVES 4 • ACTIVE TIME: 20 MINUTES • TOTAL TIME: 45 MINUTES

CAN BE MADE GLUTEN FREE, SOY FREE (LEAVE OUT THE WORCESTERSHIRE SAUCE)

I often make shepherd's pie for company, but if no one's coming over why bother with the formality of baking an actual pie? In this version, du Puy lentils and shiitake mushrooms team up to create a meaty bite. I kept the seasoning super simple, using a dash of Worcestershire sauce at the end to give the dish a little air of mystery. The nutritional info here is for the lentils only, not the potatoes, just in case you decide you'd like the lentils over rice or a baked potato or something altogether different.

2 teaspoons olive oil
1 onion, chopped finely
4 ounces shiitake mushrooms, chopped (1½ cups)
1 zucchini, diced small (1½ cups)
3 cloves garlic, minced
½ teaspoon dried tarragon
2 teaspoons dried thyme
½ teaspoon salt
   Several pinches of freshly ground black pepper
1 cup carrots, peeled and diced small
¾ cup du Puy lentils (also called French lentils), rinsed
   (see **Ingredient Scavenger Hunt**, page 199)
3 cups vegetable broth
1 tablespoon Worcestershire sauce
½ cup frozen peas
1 recipe **Caulipots** (page 54)

PER SERVING
(¼ RECIPE):
Calories: 210
Calories from fat: 15
Total fat: 2 g
Saturated fat: 0 g
Trans fat: 0 g
Total carb: 38 g
Fiber: 11 g
Sugars: 8 g
Protein: 13 g
Cholesterol: 0 mg
Sodium: 440 mg
Vitamin A: 120%
Vitamin C: 90%
Calcium: 10%
Iron: 25%

Preheat a 4-quart pot over medium-high heat. Sauté the onions in the oil until translucent, about 4 minutes. Add the shiitakes, zucchini, garlic, tarragon, thyme, salt, and pepper; sauté for 5 more minutes.

Add the carrots, lentils, and broth. Cover and bring to a boil. Once boiling, lower the heat to a simmer and cook for about 25 minutes, stirring occasionally. By this point, the lentils should be tender and most of the broth should be absorbed. If that hasn't happened yet, then cover and simmer for a bit more. Conversely, if the broth has evaporated and the lentils are not soft, then add a bit of water and simmer for a bit longer.

Once the lentils are soft, stir in the Worcestershire sauce and peas. Let sit for 10 minutes or so for maximum flavor. Taste for salt.

To serve: Scoop a cup of Caulipots into a bowl and serve a cupful of lentils over it.

∾ INGREDIENT SCAVENGER HUNT

Something's fishy. Most brands of Worcestershire sauce contain anchovies or other nonvegan ingredients, but there are quite a few vegan varieties, including Annie's, Wizard's, and Edward & Sons.

If you can't find a vegan brand in your health food store, try online at foodfightgrocery.com or CosmosVeganShoppe.com. It's a handy ingredient to have around for when you want to add a little somethin' somethin' to sauces, gravies, and bean dishes. The secret ingredient is actually tamarind.

If you can't find vegan Worcestershire, here are a few options:

If you are able to find tamarind concentrate, use 1 teaspoon of the tamarind and 2 teaspoons of soy sauce.

If you can't find any of that, use 2 teaspoons of soy sauce, 2 teaspoons of tomato paste, and 1 tablespoon of freshly squeezed lemon juice. ∾

Hottie Black-Eyed Peas & Greens

SERVES 6 • ACTIVE TIME: 20 MINUTES • TOTAL TIME: 30 MINUTES

It's hard for me to imagine having black-eyed peas without greens. They're forever linked in my taste buds, thanks to my idea of what Southerners eat every day, even though they probably eat portobellos and arugula, just like the rest of us.

Anyway, sometimes I just don't feel like using two pans. This dish works on so many levels because you don't need to sauté the greens in a ton of oil and you don't need another sauce for them; everything comes together in one pot. The vegan bar called the Bye and Bye, here in Portland, puts what I suspect is a lot of hot sauce in their black-eyed peas, so that's where this flavor profile comes from. I love to use Cholula hot sauce, but use your favorite medium-heat hot sauce (like, don't use Sriracha, but Tabasco or Frank's would be fine).

Serve with **Ginger Mashed Sweet Potatoes & Apples** (page 63), and enjoy the sweet Southern air, y'all.

- 1 teaspoon olive oil
- 1 small onion, diced small
- 2 cloves garlic, minced
- 1 bunch kale or collards, coarse stems removed, shredded (about ½ pound)
- ¼ cup water
- ¼ teaspoon salt
- 2 (15-ounce) cans black-eyed peas, drained and rinsed
- 1 cup tomato sauce
- ½ cup vegetable broth
- 1 tablespoon hot sauce
- ¼ teaspoon liquid smoke (optional; a smidge of smoked paprika would be great, too)

PER SERVING (⅙ RECIPE):
Calories: 210
Calories from fat: 15
Total fat: 2 g
Saturated fat: 0 g
Trans fat: 0 g
Total carb: 38 g
Fiber: 11 g
Sugars: 8 g
Protein: 13 g
Cholesterol: 0 mg
Sodium: 440 mg
Vitamin A: 120%
Vitamin C: 90%
Calcium: 10%
Iron: 25%

∾ **TIP** *This recipe calls for shredded greens, but all I really mean is very thinly sliced. A fast and easy way to get this done: Pile the leaves on top of each other and then roll them up. You'll see that it's very easy to slice them that way.* ∾

Preheat a 4-quart pot over medium heat. Sauté the onion in the oil until translucent, about 5 minutes. Use a little nonstick cooking spray if needed. Add the garlic and sauté for a minute more. Add the greens, 1/4 cup of water, and the salt. Cover the pot and cook down the greens for about 10 minutes, stirring occasionally. Add the black-eyed peas, tomato sauce, and broth, and mix thoroughly. Cover the pot and cook for about 5 minutes, stirring occasionally.

Add the hot sauce and liquid smoke, then use a potato masher to mash some of the beans, about one-quarter of them, to thicken the sauce. Cook for about 5 more minutes, uncovered. Taste for salt and seasoning. You may want to add more hot sauce.

∾ NUTRITION TIP *Peas and greens are a wonderful combination for taste and nutrition. With one serving you will eat as much fiber as the average American gets in a whole day! Plus a day's worth of vitamin A and a quarter of the iron. Combine with one serving of the Ginger Mashed Sweet Potatoes and Apples, and you'll have 16 grams of protein and nearly one-fifth of your calcium for the day. All with only 2 grams of fat and less than 400 calories.* ∾

Baked Falafel

MAKES 12 FALAFEL, SERVES 4 • ACTIVE TIME: 20 MINUTES • TOTAL TIME: 45 MINUTES

Of course, we all love deep-fried foods, but so long as your falafel has plenty of flavor, it won't lose too much in the low-fat baked translation. My version uses pureed chickpeas, as well as a little chickpea flour to give it extra of that savory chickpea flavor. I love fresh herbs in falafel, Israeli style. Use either flat-leaf parsley or cilantro; it's all up to your personal preference.

When baking falafel, it works best to form them into patties instead of balls; that way they cook evenly. I forgo the traditional pita because I love to serve them over salad, especially arugula, sprinkled with a little freshly squeezed lemon juice and coarsely ground kosher salt. You can also pile on the veggies; tomatoes, cucumber and red onion are all natural choices. Any variation on the hummus makes a great accompaniment, so go ahead and double your chickpea pleasure.

And if you would like pita, there are some wonderful whole wheat brands on the market, and even whole wheat mini pitas. But if you're looking for something lighter, try making a lettuce wrap instead.

1	(15-ounce) can chickpeas, drained and rinsed
2	cloves garlic
½	small white onion, chopped roughly (about 3 tablespoons)
½	cup loosely packed fresh parsley leaves
2	teaspoons olive oil
2	teaspoons hot sauce
3 to 4	tablespoons chickpea flour
1	teaspoon ground cumin
1	teaspoon ground coriander
½	teaspoon paprika
½	teaspoon baking powder
¼	teaspoon salt, or to taste
	Several pinches of freshly ground black pepper

PER SERVING
(¼ RECIPE, FALAFEL INGREDIENTS ONLY):
Calories: 140
Calories from fat: 40
Total fat: 4.5 g
Saturated fat: 0 g
Trans fat: 0 g
Total carb: 19 g
Fiber: 5 g
Sugars: 3 g
Protein: 6 g
Cholesterol: 0 mg
Sodium: 380 mg
Vitamin A: 15%
Vitamin C: 25%
Calcium: 10%
Iron: 15%

TIP *These make a great packed lunch! I think they taste best at room temp, so store in the fridge until about an hour before you eat, then leave out at room temp, just to take the chill off.*

Arugula or other salad greens

Chopped or sliced tomato

Diced or sliced cucumber

Sliced red onion

Lemon wedges

Chopped fresh parsley or cilantro

Kosher salt

Preheat the oven to 400°F.

Pulse the chickpeas and garlic in a food processor. Add the onion, parley, olive oil, and hot sauce, and blend until relatively smooth, scraping down the sides if necessary to make sure you get everything.

Transfer the mixture to a mixing bowl. Mix in the 3 tablespoons of chickpea flour, cumin, coriander, paprika, baking powder, salt, and pepper. The mixture should be mushy but firm enough to shape into balls. If it doesn't seem firm enough, add a tablespoon of chickpea flour.

Spray a baking sheet with nonstick cooking spray. Form the mixture into walnut-size balls, then flatten a bit into patties. Place on the baking sheet. Bake for 16 to 18 minutes; they should be browned on the underside. Remove the falafel from the oven, spray them with a little cooking spray, then flip the falafel and bake for 8 to 10 more minutes.

They're now ready to serve; try some of the suggestions above.

ॐ INGREDIENT SCAVENGER HUNT

Chickpea flour, also known as garbanzo flour or simply as besan in the Indian culinary world, is just what it sounds like: ground, dried chickpeas. It's easy to find in the gluten-free section of most well-stocked supermarkets; a popular brand is Bob's Red Mill. They also make a garbanzo-fava blend that would work just fine, also available in many Indian and Israeli markets. If you absolutely cannot or do not want to use it in this recipe, regular old flour will work just fine. ॐ

Chipotle Lentil Burgers

MAKES 6 BURGERS • ACTIVE TIME: 30 MINUTES • TOTAL TIME: 30 MINUTES

Burgers with a smoky, spicy kick! Serve these topped with your favorite salsa alongside some **OMG Oven-Baked Onion Rings** (page 59). Or, if you want some added heat, smash up a chipotle in ¼ cup of ketchup. These have a firm, bready exterior and a softer interior; they're not trying to replicate meat, they're veggie burgers! Lots of recipes in this book aren't finicky, but this one you need to follow to the letter. To get the texture right you have to use store-bought bread crumbs and canned lentils; otherwise you'll be messing with the dry and wet ingredient ratio too much.

PER SERVING
(⅙ RECIPE):
Calories: 130
Calories from fat: 15
Total fat: 1.5 g
Saturated fat: 0 g
Trans fat: 0 g
Total carb: 23 g
Fiber: 7 g
Sugars: 3 g
Protein: 8 g
Cholesterol: 0 mg
Sodium: 510 mg
Vitamin A: 15%
Vitamin C: 20%
Calcium: 4%
Iron: 20%

- 1 teaspoon olive oil
- 1 small red onion, cut into medium dice
- ½ pound zucchini, halved lengthwise and sliced ½ inch thick
- 3 cloves garlic, minced
- 1 cup lightly packed fresh cilantro, chopped (stems and leaves)
- 1 (15-ounce) can cooked lentils, drained and rinsed (1¼ cups)
- 1 cup bread crumbs
- ¼ cup chipotles, seeds removed, with adobe sauce
- 2 tablespoons soy sauce
- 2 teaspoons red wine vinegar
- ¼ teaspoon salt
- 2 teaspoons smoked paprika

First, we're going to sauté some veggies. Preheat a large, heavy-bottomed nonstick pan, preferably cast iron, over medium-high heat. Sauté the onion for about 3 minutes. Add the zucchini, garlic, cilantro, and a pinch of salt, and sauté for 7 to 10 minutes, until the zucchini is soft.

Transfer the zucchini mixture to a food processor. Add all the other ingredients except for ½ cup of the bread crumbs. Did you hear me? Reserve ½ cup of the bread crumbs! Pulse until mostly smooth, but there should still be a little texture. Transfer to a large mixing bowl.

> ∾ **TIP** *To get these done in a half-hour, assemble everything else while the zucchini is cooking.* ∾

Preheat the pan (the same one you already used to sauté in is fine) over medium heat. Add the remaining ½ cup of bread crumbs to the burger mixture and use a fork to thoroughly combine.

Divide the burger mixture into six equal pieces. An easy way to do this is divide it in half, then divide each half into three basically equal portions. You can do that right in the mixing bowl if it's large enough.

Spray the pan with nonstick cooking spray. Form the burger portions into patties (see tip) and cook for about 12 minutes, flipping the burgers often, until they are nicely browned on both sides. Use cooking spray as necessary. Do three at a time for best results.

They taste great served immediately but they're also excellent at room temperature, so don't be afraid to stuff one into a sandwich and take it for lunch.

> ∾ TIP Don't be too OCD about getting the seeds out of the chipotles, just do your best. The more seeds there are the spicier this will be, so I prefer to remove them so I can use more of the chipotles and get more flavor without burning off my beautiful face. ∾

> ∾ INGREDIENT SCAVENGER HUNT
> Precooked lentils aren't all that common yet, but their presence on the shelves is growing! If you can't find them at your regular old supermarket, Whole Foods Market or Trader Joe's will probably carry them. ∾

> ∾ TIP For perfectly shaped burgers, get yourself a sheet of parchment paper. Put a 3-inch round cookie cutter on the parchment, spray with nonstick cooking spray, and place your veggie burger in there to mold it. Lift the cookie cutter and voilà!—a veggie burger that looks like it's on TV. Lifestyles of the Rich and Famous, to be exact. ∾

Forty-Clove Chickpeas & Broccoli

SERVES 4 • ACTIVE TIME: 15 MINUTES • TOTAL TIME: 50 MINUTES

Okay, there aren't really forty cloves of garlic here, I just always liked how 40-Clove Chicken sounded. But there *are* ten and that's still a lot! The idea of this recipe is to chop up your brocs and have everything in the oven within 15 minutes and then go start your *Trapper John, MD* marathon, paint your toenails, and check on the food every once in a while. When it does come out of the oven, you'll have a scrumptious garlicky meal, complete with tender (but not mushy) roasted broccoli and chickpeas that turn deliciously creamy (but not mushy!). The garlic should turn tender and creamy as well, and its flavor will mellow and sweeten.

It's nothing fancy, don't serve it to your in-laws, but when I'm just hanging out and desperately need something healthy with hardly any effort, then many a night I've thrown this together.

PER SERVING
(¼ RECIPE):
Calories: 170
Calories from fat: 40
Total fat: 4.5 g
Saturated fat: 0 g
Trans fat: 0 g
Total carb: 27 g
Fiber: 8 g
Sugars: 5 g
Protein: 9 g
Cholesterol: 0 mg
Sodium: 590 mg
Vitamin A: 15%
Vitamin C: 180%
Calcium: 10%
Iron: 15%

- 1 pound broccoli, cut into large spears, stems chopped in ½-inch pieces
- 10 cloves garlic, smashed (see tip)
- 1 (15-ounce) can chickpeas, drained and rinsed
- 2 teaspoons olive oil
- ½ teaspoon salt
  Freshly ground black pepper
- 2 teaspoons lemon zest
- 1½ teaspoons dried oregano
- 1 cup vegetable broth

> **NUTRITION TIP** *Garlic contains allyl sulfides, phytochemicals that may play a role in protection against heart disease and cancer, among other health benefits.*

Preheat the oven to 400°F. Place the broccoli, garlic, and chickpeas in a 9 by 13-inch baking pan. Drizzle them with oil, spray with a little nonstick cooking spray, and toss to coat. Sprinkle with the salt, several pinches of pepper, and the lemon zest and oregano. Once again, toss to coat. Spray a bit more for good measure, then pop it in the oven.

Bake for about 30 minutes, flipping once. Remove from the oven, flip again, and add the vegetable broth. Use a spatula to scrape up any crisp bits of flavor from the bottom on the pan. Return the pan to the oven for another 15 minutes, or until the garlic cloves are nice and tender and the broccoli is browned in some places.

> ∽ TIP *The cloves of garlic should remain relatively whole. To smash them, break the garlic into individual cloves, then on a hard surface lay your knife flat against the garlic and give your knife a whack. The skin should become loose. Just peel it off and there's your smashed garlic. Sometimes the clove breaks up more, sometimes less, but for this recipe anything goes.* ∽

Mushroom & Cannellini Paprikas

SERVES 4 • ACTIVE TIME: 20 MINUTES • TOTAL TIME: 30 MINUTES

(CAN BE MADE GLUTEN FREE IF SERVED ON ITS OWN OR WITH CAULIPOTS)

When I think of a dish that's traditionally meaty and I don't want to use the holy trinity (tempeh, tofu, and seitan), I usually reach for mushrooms. This dish is a perfect example. Mushrooms, wine, and garlic will have you reliving your Hungarian childhood. Make sure to get the smoked variety of paprika for that added depth of flavor. Serve over **Scarlet Barley** (page 69) or **Caulipots** (page 54).

1½ teaspoons olive oil
 Small red onion, sliced thinly (about 1 cup)
 4 cloves garlic, minced
 1 pound cremini mushrooms, sliced
 Several pinches of freshly ground black pepper
 ¼ teaspoon salt
 ½ cup dry red cooking wine
 ¼ cup vegetable broth
 2 teaspoons smoked paprika
 2 tablespoons fresh chopped thyme
 1 (16-ounce) can cannellini beans, drained and rinsed
 ¼ cup chopped fresh dill
 1 recipe Scarlet Barley or Caulipots (to serve)

Preheat a 4-quart pot over medium-high heat. Sauté the onions in the oil until lightly browned, about 7 minutes. Add the garlic and sauté for about 30 seconds. Add the mushrooms, pepper, and salt; cook until lots of the moisture has been released, stirring occasionally, for about 5 minutes.

Add the wine, broth, smoked paprika, and thyme. Turn up the heat and bring the mixture to a low boil. Boil for about 3 minutes. Lower the

PER SERVING
(¼ RECIPE):
Calories: 170
Calories from fat: 20
Total fat: 2.5 g
Saturated fat: 0 g
Trans fat: 0 g
Total carb: 27 g
Fiber: 7 g
Sugars: 5 g
Protein: 11 g
Cholesterol: 0 mg
Sodium: 490 g
Vitamin A: 10%
Vitamin C: 15%
Calcium: 8%
Iron: 15%

heat and add the beans. Cook to heat through, about 5 more minutes. Use a strong fork to lightly mash some of the beans, to thicken the sauce. Just mash a few against the side of the pot and then mix 'em back in. Taste for salt and serve.

Serve over Scarlet Barley or Caulipots and litter with plenty of fresh dill.

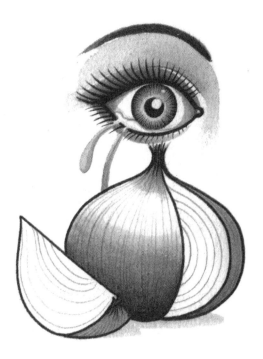

Caribbean Curried Black-Eyed Peas with Plantains

SERVES 4 • ACTIVE TIME: 20 MINUTES • TOTAL TIME: 30 MINUTES

In my old neighborhood in Brooklyn, the streets were lined with spicy, sexy, West Indian curries. I really miss the tropical flavors, but I don't miss the feeling of eating a small army's ration of coconut milk. And those deep-fried plantains were killer, but they probably *will* kill you someday. In this revamped dish, just a touch of coconut milk really does the job, and steaming the plantains coaxes out their sweet flavor and succulent texture even better than frying does.

Jamaican curries were influenced by Indian curries, but with their own spin on the spice blend. The biggest difference is that Jamaican curry powder calls for star anise. Because preblended Jamaican curry powder can be hard to find, I rigged up this cheater blend simply by adding star anise to a regular old curry powder. Serve with brown basmati rice or **Mashed Yuca with Cilantro & Lime** (page 57) and **Jerk Asparagus** (page 91).

PER SERVING
(¼ RECIPE):
Calories: 300
Calories from fat: 45
Total fat: 5 g
Saturated fat: 2.5 g
Trans fat: 0 g
Total carb: 57 g
Fiber: 10 g
Sugars: 18 g
Protein: 11 g
Cholesterol: 0 mg
Sodium: 320 mg
Vitamin A: 25%
Vitamin C: 40%
Calcium: 6%
Iron: 25%

- 1 teaspoon olive oil
- ¼ cup finely chopped shallot
- 1 red bell pepper, seeded and diced finely
- ½ to 1 habanero pepper, seeded and minced
- 3 cloves garlic, minced
- 2 teaspoons minced fresh ginger
- 2 bay leaves
- 1 star anise
- 2 teaspoons mild curry powder
- Pinch of ground cinnamon
- About 3 sprigs of fresh thyme
- ½ teaspoon salt
- ¾ cup light coconut milk
- ¾ cup water
- 1 (16-ounce) can black-eyed peas, drained and rinsed

⁓ TIP

Habanero peppers are really hot, so proceed with caution. If you're not absolutely crazy about spicy food, do half a habanero. Or for even milder flavor, use half a jalapeño pepper. ⁓

1 teaspoon light agave nectar
  Juice from about ½ lime
2 very ripe plantains, split lengthwise and cut into 1-inch chunks
  Cooked rice or other grain, for serving

Bring your steamer apparatus to a boil and preheat a small, heavy-bottomed pot over medium heat. Sauté the shallot, red pepper, and habanero in the oil for about 5 minutes, until softened. Add the garlic, ginger, bay leaves, and star anise, and sauté for about 2 minutes more. Add a splash of water and the curry powder, cinnamon, and thyme. Stir for about 30 seconds, just to toast the curry powder a bit.

Add the salt, coconut milk, water, and beans. Cover and heat through for about 5 minutes. Add the agave and lime. Taste for salt and seasoning. Turn off the heat and let the curry sit for 10 minutes to allow the flavors to meld. Remove the thyme, anise, and bay leaves.

In the meantime, steam the plantains for about 5 minutes. They should appear plump and bright yellow.

To assemble: Serve the beans over rice (or any grain) in wide, rimmed bowls. Top with the plantains.

∿ INGREDIENT SCAVENGER HUNT

Plantains are a tropical fruit that look like big bananas, but their texture is firmer and more starchy, so they're a better fit for savory food than for desserts. Many supermarkets carry plantains, but you might have better luck at a West Indian, South Asian, or Latin market. If you can't find plantains for the life of you, then steam a big sweet potato for this dish. Peel and cut into ½-inch pieces, and steam for about 10 minutes. It'll give you the touch of sweetness this recipe is looking for. ∿

Black Bean, Zucchini, & Olive Tacos

MAKES 8 TACOS • ACTIVE TIME: 20 MINUTES • TOTAL TIME: 25 MINUTES

Have you got some zucchini burning a hole in your pocket? These tacos should do the trick. Tacos somehow *sound* unhealthy, but they aren't. Corn tortillas are low in fat and have some fiber, too. The key, I think, is to make the filling somewhat saucy and packed with flavor, so that a bunch of guac and cheese is not needed.

Olives are often overlooked in Latin foods, but they work so well, adding bursts of succulent, salty flavor. Here I use canned tomatillos (salsa verde) to make for a superfast weeknight meal and chopped kalamata olives for a burst of salty flavor. You can serve with the Garlic-Lemon Yogurt, but it's not wholly necessary; I eat these all by their lonesome all the time. If you've got some fresh greens to add, you can go ahead and do that, too.

1 teaspoon olive oil
2 zucchini, diced small (about 1 pound)
2 jalapeños, seeded, sliced thinly
¼ teaspoon salt
2 cloves garlic, minced
⅓ cup pitted kalamata olives, chopped
½ teaspoon ground cumin
½ teaspoon ground coriander
1 (6-ounce) can salsa verde
1 (16-ounce) can black beans, drained and rinsed
½ cup finely chopped scallions
8 (6-inch) corn tortillas

PER SERVING
(1 TACO; ⅛ RECIPE):
Calories: 160
Calories from fat: 25
Total fat: 2.5 g
Saturated fat: 0 g
Trans fat: 0 g
Total carb: 29 g
Fiber: 8 g
Sugars: 2 g
Protein: 7 g
Cholesterol: 0 mg
Sodium: 290 mg
Vitamin A: 4%
Vitamin C: 25%
Calcium: 6%
Iron: 10%

∾ INGREDIENT SCAVENGER HUNT

You should be able to find a small can of salsa verde in the Latin aisle of your supermarket. It shouldn't contain many more ingredients than tomatillo, jalapeño, cilantro, and salt. ∾

Preheat a heavy-bottomed skillet over medium-high heat. Add the zucchini and jalapeño to the oil and sprinkle with the salt (salt will help draw the moisture out of the zukes). Sauté for about 7 minutes, until the zucchini is lightly browned. Add the garlic, olives, cumin, and coriander, and sauté for 2 minutes more.

Add the salsa verde and black beans. Cook for 5 more minutes; the salsa should reduce a bit so that it's juicy but not soupy.

Place the tortillas in a moist paper towel and heat in the microwave for 1 minute on high. Serve with Garlic-Lemon Yogurt and chopped scallions.

Garlic–Lemon Yogurt

1	cup unsweetened plain yogurt (Wildwood is great)
2 to 3	cloves garlic
	Zest from ½ lemon
	Juice from 1 lemon (about 3 tablespoons)
½	teaspoon light agave nectar

PER SERVING
(1 TABLESPOON):
The nutritional information is included in the tacos list.

Scoop the yogurt into a small bowl. Use a Microplane to grate in the garlic and then the lemon zest. Squeeze in the lemon juice and add the agave. Use a fork to mix well. Taste and adjust the garlic and lemon to your liking.

Mango BBQ Beans

SERVES 6 • ACTIVE TIME: 15 MINUTES • TOTAL TIME: 1 HOUR

Plain old BBQ beans are nice and everything, but mango gives them another dimension—a tart, tropical sweetness that makes them a bit more special. Barbecue flavors really benefit from a nice, long cooking time. Let these simmer on the stove for at least 45 minutes so that the beans absorb more of the flavor and the mango cooks down and melds with the tomato sauce. Serve with greens and rice, with a piece of **Fresh Corn & Scallion Corn Bread** (page 244), or over **Mashed Yuca with Cilantro & Lime** (page 57).

PER SERVING
(⅙ RECIPE):
Calories: 220
Calories from fat: 15
Total fat: 1.5 g
Saturated fat: 0 g
Trans fat: 0 g
Total carb: 43 g
Fiber: 9 g
Sugars: 13 g
Protein: 12 g
Cholesterol: 0 mg
Sodium: 480 mg
Vitamin A: 8%
Vitamin C: 25%
Calcium: 6%
Iron: 20%

- 1 teaspoon olive oil
- 1 onion, chopped finely
- 3 cloves garlic, minced
- 1 mango, seeded and chopped small
- 1 cup tomato sauce
- 1 cup vegetable broth
- ½ teaspoon red pepper flakes, or ¼ teaspoon if you want it less spicy
- ¼ teaspoon allspice
- 1 teaspoon ground coriander
- ½ teaspoon salt
- 1 (25-ounce) can kidney beans, drained and rinsed
- 1 teaspoon liquid smoke
- 2 to 3 tablespoons agave nectar

Preheat a 4-quart pot over medium heat. Sauté the onion and garlic in the oil with a pinch of salt for about 5 minutes, until translucent.

Add the mango, tomato sauce, broth, red pepper flakes, coriander, salt, and kidney beans. Turn up the heat and bring to a rolling boil. Lower the heat to a simmer and cover the pot, leaving a little room for steam to escape, and let cook for about 45 minutes, stirring often. The sauce should thicken and the mangoes should cook down a great deal.

Turn off the heat, mix in the agave and liquid smoke, and let the beans sit for about 5 minutes. Taste for sweetness and add more agave if needed. Adjust the salt and seasonings, and serve.

Black Beans in Red Velvet Mole

SERVES 6 • ACTIVE TIME: 20 MINUTES • TOTAL TIME: 30 MINUTES

PER SERVING
(⅙ RECIPE):
Calories: 270
Calories from fat: 35
Total fat: 4 g
Saturated fat: 0.5 g
Trans fat: 0 g
Total carb: 49 mg
Fiber: 13 g
Sugars: 14 g
Protein: 13 g
Cholesterol: 0 mg
Sodium: 140 mg
Vitamin A: 30%
Vitamin C: 25%
Calcium: 10%
Iron: 20%

Black beans in a rich, smoky *mole rojo*. All the layers of flavor you expect from mole are here: chocolate, chili, tomato, and a bit of sweetness from raisins and anise. Tortilla chips bring lots of body and flavor, and a touch of cinnamon brings warmth that just begs to top off roasted pumpkin, or try it with the **Ginger Mashed Sweet Potatoes & Apples** (page 63). I just think a hint of sweetness sets things off nicely, so even if you're serving over brown rice, add some steamed plantains. I'm listing the sauce separately because it's great for pouring over roasted veggies or Latin-inspired bowls. Use whatever almond or peanut butter you have on hand for this.

RED VELVET MOLE:

- 1 teaspoon olive oil
- 1 small onion, cut into medium dice
- 3 cloves garlic, minced
- 1 teaspoon aniseeds
- 5 teaspoons chili powder
- 2 teaspoons dried oregano or marjoram
- 1 teaspoon ground cinnamon
- ¼ teaspoon ground allspice
- 1 teaspoon smoked paprika
- 1 (16-ounce) can diced tomatoes
- 1 cup vegetable broth
- ¼ cup raisins
- ¼ cup crushed low-fat tortilla chips
- 3 tablespoons unsweetened cocoa powder
- 1 tablespoon almond or peanut butter
- 2 tablespoons agave nectar
- 1 (24-ounce) can black beans, drained and rinsed

Preheat a 2-quart pot over medium heat. Sauté the onion in the oil for 5 to 7 minutes, until translucent. Add the garlic, herbs, and spices. Sauté for another minute or so.

Add the tomatoes and broth, and bring to a boil. Once boiling, add the raisins, tortilla chips, chocolate powder, and almond butter. Simmer for about 15 minutes, until slightly reduced.

Once the mole has cooked for 15 minutes, use a submersion blender to puree it smooth. If you don't have a submersion blender, transfer it to the food processor or blender and puree until smooth. If your blender isn't equipped with a lid that has an opening on top, make sure to lift the lid every few seconds so that the steam doesn't build up and kill you.

Transfer the mole back to the pot and stir in the agave. Taste for seasonings and add the beans. Let sit for at least 10 minutes so that the flavors "marry." Taste and adjust the seasoning if necessary.

Unfried Refried Beans

SERVES 6 • ACTIVE TIME: 10 MINUTES • TOTAL TIME: 20 MINUTES

Refried beans aren't actually beans that are fried twice, they're beans that have been very well fried. These refried beans, however, are neither twice fried nor well fried; they're completely unfried. I use tomato sauce to get that mouthwatering consistency you've come to expect from refried beans, without using that ½ cup of oil you've come to regret. This is one of those recipes I've been making forever; it's completely dependable in tacos or over rice, when you get that hankering for a Mexican-inspired meal but don't want to spend a lot of time.

> 1 teaspoon extra-virgin olive oil
> 1 small yellow onion, chopped finely
> 3 cloves garlic, minced
> 1 tablespoon coriander seeds, crushed (see tip, page 220)
> 2 teaspoons ground cumin
> ½ teaspoon salt
> 1 (24-ounce) can pinto beans, drained and rinsed
> 1 (8-ounce) can tomato sauce
>   Pinch of cayenne (optional)

Preheat a 2-quart pot over medium heat. Sauté the onion in the oil for 3 to 5 minutes, until translucent. Add the garlic, coriander, cumin, and salt. Sauté for another minute or so. Use splashes of water if it appears dry.

Add the pinto beans and mash with a fork or a mini-potato masher (or avocado masher). Add the tomato sauce and mix well. Cook to heat through, adding splashes of water to thin, if necessary. If you like it spicy, mix in a pinch of cayenne.

Hummus & Friends

SERVES 8 (ABOUT ¼-CUP EACH) • TIME: 10 MINUTES

The secret to great-tasting and creamy low-fat hummus is to reserve a little bit of the chickpea liquid. This oil-free hummus might not be the one I would take to a potluck to impress people, but if I'm settling in for a night of TV and want to mindlessly munch on some carrot sticks, this dip really does the trick. It's also wonderful over the **Baked Falafel** (page 121), or to top off a salad. I love that you can eat this in ¼-cup servings, or heck, have a little more if you want! I laugh at the serving size of those nutrition labels in the supermarket because really, who eats just a tablespoon of hummus?

BASIC RECIPE:

- 1 (15-ounce) can chickpeas, liquid reserved
- 2 cloves garlic
- 1 tablespoon olive oil
- 2 tablespoons freshly squeezed lemon juice
- ¼ teaspoon salt
- ½ teaspoon paprika (optional)

When you open the can of chickpeas, pour about 3 tablespoons of the liquid into a cup and set aside. Drain the rest of the liquid and rinse the chickpeas. Pulse them in a food processor along with the garlic until no whole chickpeas are left. Add the olive oil and lemon juice and puree for a bit. Add 2 tablespoons of the reserved liquid, the salt, and paprika, if using. Blend until very smooth, adding the last tablespoon of liquid if needed. Scrape down the sides of the food processor with a spatula to make sure you get everything. Taste for salt and lemon juice. You can serve immediately, but I like to let it chill for at least an hour.

PER SERVING
(⅛ OF RECIPE)
Calories: 60
Calories from fat: 20
Total fat: 2.5 g
Saturated fat: 0 g
Trans fat: 0 g
Total carb: 9 g
Fiber: 2 g
Sugars: <1 g
Protein: 4 g
Cholesterol: 0 mg
Sodium: 260 mg
Vitamin A: 0%
Vitamin C: 4%
Calcium: 0%
Iron: 4%

And now for the friends!

Horseradish-Dill Hummus

1 tablespoon prepared horseradish
¼ cup loosely packed fresh dill

Puree the horseradish along with everything else. Pulse in the dill until chopped finely.

PER SERVING (⅛ OF RECIPE) Adds 1 g of sugar and 2% Vitamin C to the Hummus nutritional info in the main recipe.

Curried Green Onion Hummus

2 to 3 teaspoons curry powder
½ cup chopped green onions

Puree the curry powder along with everything else. Pulse in the green onions until chopped finely.

PER SERVING (⅛ OF RECIPE) Adds 2% calcium to the Hummus nutritional info in the main recipe.

Shabby Sheik Hummus

1 teaspoon ground cumin
1 teaspoon smoked paprika
¼ teaspoon cayenne

Puree the spices along with other ingredients in the hummus.

PER SERVING (⅛ OF RECIPE) The nutritional info is the same as for the main recipe.

Roasted Red Pepper & Kalamata Hummus

1   roasted red pepper, peeled and seeded (¼ cup if from a jar)
¼   cup pitted kalamata olives

Puree the red pepper along with everything else. Pulse in the olives until chopped finely.

PER SERVING (⅛ OF RECIPE) Adds 10 calories, 10 calories from fat, .5 g total fat, 2g carbs, 1 g fiber, 2 g sugar, 80 mg niacin, 10 % vitamin A, and 31 % vitamin C to the Hummus nutritional info in the main recipe.

Pizza Hummus

¼   cup chopped sun-dried tomatoes (not oil-packed)
1   cup fresh basil

Reconstitute the tomatoes in a bowl by submerging them in warm water for about 15 minutes. Puree along with everything else. Pulse in the basil until chopped finely.

PER SERVING (⅛ OF RECIPE) The nutritional info is the same as for the main recipe.

Jalapeño-Cilantro Hummus

1   seeded, chopped average sized jalapeno
½   cup fresh cilantro

After pureeing, pulse the jalapeño and cilantro into the hummus until chopped finely.

PER SERVING (⅛ OF RECIPE) Adds .5 g fiber, less than 1 g sugar, 2% vitamin A, 2% vitamin C, and 2% calcium to the Hummus nutritional info in the main recipe.

CHAPTER 5

Sink-Your-Teeth-Into Tofu & Tempeh

TOFU IS LIKE THAT FRIEND WHO ALWAYS KNOWS EXACTLY WHAT to say. So versatile and accomodating, tofu is there when you need her. Breakfast? Sure, try a scramble. Lunch? How about baked and sliced in sandwiches? And for dinner, whether it be a fancy night out on the town or a quiet evening at home with a *Law & Order* marathon, tofu knows what's up.

If tofu is the fun-loving soy next door, tempeh is its more grown-up cousin. Tempeh is a soy patty, but that description doesn't exactly get the tongues wagging. It's from Indonesia, and has a rich and interesting history, but really, all of that info can be Googled.

The reason I love tempeh is because the first time I tasted it, in burger form at a vegan restaurant in the '80s, it was so delicious it made my eyes roll back in my head. I had only been vegetarian for a short while, but sinking my teeth into that tempeh, I knew I was gonna be all right. It was downright succulent and the flavor complex—nutty, earthy, meaty. Everything you could want out of food.

Together, tofu and tempeh are true Wonder Twins. Topping salads or mashed potatoes and fighting crime, soy can do it all deliciously.

The Great Soy Scare

There's a lot of scare mongering (soy mongering?) all over the place lately. I asked Matt to clear up some misconceptions about soy and here is what he had to say. He even cited a few sources to make it easier for you to do your own research and fact checking!

Soybeans have been a part of people's diets for thousands of years. It's a bean, so it's full of plant protein, healthy fats, and phytochemicals. In the last thirty years we've seen a lot of research on its ability to reduce cholesterol, lower cancer risk, and possibly even help prevent obesity.[1]

After the FDA approved the statement that soy is healthy for your heart,[2] even more research came out. We are talking dozens of studies in research journals every month. Food companies jumped on the soy bandwagon and started putting it in everything from potato chips to pasta. Soon enough the backlash came, challenging it as a "superfood." I hate to say *smear campaign*, but suddenly antisoy propaganda appeared everywhere. "It's unsafe for kids!" "There's estrogen in it, so it gives men boobs!" None of this is true.[3] There is no estrogen in soy like the estrogen our body produces, thankfully. Some of the phytochemicals have the unfortunate name of phytoestrogens, but they act against estrogen mostly and are the compounds that have the benefits!

The research says that soy is safe for everyone. People have been eating it for a long time and the people who eat the most it have lower rates of cancer[4] and heart disease, even when we take other factors into consideration. Try to eat it in its most whole form—think more edamame and less textured vegetable protein. And don't worry about your sperm count decreasing or your breasts growing because of a simple bean. That just doesn't happen!

---

1. A. Ørgaard and L. Jensen, "The Effects of Soy Isoflavones on Obesity," *Experimental Biology and Medicine* 233 (2008):1066–1080.

2. Food and Drug Administration, "Food Labeling: Health Claims; Soy Protein and Coronary Heart Disease" *Federal Register* (October 26, 1999), http://www.federalregister.gov/articles/1999/10/26/99-27693/food-labeling-health-claims-soy-protein-and-coronary-heart-disease.

3. J. M. Hamilton-Reeves, G. Vazquez, et al. "Clinical Studies Show No Effects of Soy Protein or Isoflavones on Reproductive Hormones in Men: Results of a Meta-Analysis," *Fertility and Sterility* (June 11, 2009).

4. L. A. Korde, A. H. Wu, et al., "Childhood Soy Intake and Breast Cancer Risk in Asian American Women," *Cancer Epidemiology, Biomarkers & Prevention* (April 18, 2009):1050.

Tofu & Tempeh in Training

Some of these recipes assume you know a couple of things about tofu, but just in case you don't, here is where you report for tofu basic training.

HOW TO PRESS TOFU (AND WHY, FOR GOODNESS' SAKE?)

With the exception of a few brands, extra-firm tofu, the kind I most often call for, usually comes packed in water. If you would like your tofu to absorb more flavor, you press it first to get rid of some of the water and make room for more marinade. There are expensive tofu-pressing gadgets out there, but really, all you need are a flat surface, a clean kitchen towel, and a really heavy book. You can also add a couple of cans of beans for good measure.

Remove the tofu from the package and press it lightly with your hands over the sink to remove some of the water. Wrap it in a kitchen towel and set it on a counter. Balance a superheavy, hardcover book on the tofu. Place a few cans of beans on the book. Let the tofu rest for half an hour, then flip and press for another half hour. Change the kitchen towel if it appears excessively soaked. Your tofu is now pressed and ready to use!

HOW TO TAME YOUR TEMPEH

Tempeh can have a bitter flavor, but not necessarily in a bad way, more like in an arugula way. If you're easing into the world of tempeh, have something against arugula, or just want the other flavors you're using to stand out more, steaming the tempeh is the way to go. First slice the tempeh into the desired shape, then steam for about 10 minutes. Another benefit of steaming is that it loosens up the tempeh and gets it ready to soak up more marinade. Can't go wrong there.

Basic Baked Tofu (or Tempeh)

SERVES 4 • ACTIVE TIME: 10 MINUTES • TOTAL TIME: 2 HOURS

(CAN BE MADE GLUTEN FREE IF USING GF TAMARI)

~~~~~~~~~~~~~~~

PER SERVING
(¼ RECIPE):
Calories: 90
Calories from fat: 35
Total fat: 4 g
Saturated fat: 1 g
Trans fat: 0 g
Total carb: 5 g
Fiber: <1 g
Sugars: 2 g
Protein: 9 g
Cholesterol: 0 mg
Sodium: 500 mg
Vitamin A: 0%
Vitamin C: 0%
Calcium: 20%
Iron: 10%

Basic. Like black jeans and a hoodie and flip-flops and that messenger bag you've had since the Clinton administration. Well, maybe your basic is a little different, but this tofu is pretty ubiquitous. Any health food store in the United States will carry a tofu like this, perfect for tucking into sandwiches, topping salads, or serving as a main dish along with some **Caulipots** (page 54), greens, and gravy. The nutritional info is for two slices, but the serving size really depends what you're using it for. For example, maybe you want to slice off one piece to top a salad, but use three slices in a sandwich.

Back when I had an office job, I'd make the marinade the night before and press the tofu when I woke up. I'd get ready, put on my face and all that, then put the tofu in the marinade for the day. You don't get to flip it, but if it's mostly submerged that shouldn't be too much of a problem.

MARINADE:
- ¾ cup vegetable broth
- 3 tablespoons balsamic vinegar
- 2 tablespoons tamari or soy sauce
- 1 teaspoon dried thyme
- 3 cloves garlic, minced

TOFU:
- 1 block extra-firm tofu (about 14 ounces), pressed

Prepare the marinade by combining all its ingredients in a wide, shallow bowl.

Cut the tofu widthwise into eight equal pieces. If you like, slice those pieces corner to corner to form triangles. Marinate for at least an hour, flipping after 30 minutes.

Preheat the oven to 375°F. Spray a baking sheet with nonstick cooking spray. Place the tofu on the baking sheet and bake for 20 minutes. Spray with a little more cooking spray and flip the pieces. Spoon some marinade over each piece and bake for another 10 minutes. If you like, place under the broiler for about 3 more minutes, for extra chewiness.

~~~~~~

Variation: Basic Baked Tempeh

Mix together the marinade ingredients and marinate the tempeh for at least an hour, or up to overnight.

Preheat the oven to 400°F. Lightly oil a baking sheet. Place the tempeh slices in a single layer on the baking sheet. Bake for 25 to 30 minutes, flipping once. Spoon extra marinade over the tempeh a few times during baking.

Masala Baked Tofu

SERVES 4 • ACTIVE TIME: 10 MINUTES • TOTAL TIME: 2 HOURS

G **D**

(CAN BE MADE GLUTEN FREE IF USING GF TAMARI)

It's pretty obvious that this will go with all the Indian-inspired dishes, but I really like to put this tofu where it doesn't belong—on top of **Pasta con Broccoli** (page 169), inside the **Black Bean, Zucchini, & Olive Tacos** (page 131) or on a salad with **Carrot–Ginger Dressing** (page 52). Vegan food can be a clash of food and culture, so think outside the tofu box and have some fun. You can also just make a sandwich out of this, with some hummus or reduced-fat mayo and the usual suspects, lettuce, tomato, and onion.

MARINADE:

¾ cup vegetable broth

2 tablespoons rice vinegar

2 tablespoons tamari or soy sauce

2 tablespoons curry powder

3 cloves garlic, minced

2 teaspoons minced fresh ginger

TOFU:

1 block extra-firm tofu (about 14 ounces), pressed

Prepare the marinade by combining all its ingredients in a wide, shallow bowl.

Cut the tofu widthwise into eight equal pieces. If you like, slice those pieces corner to corner to form triangles. Marinate for at least an hour, or up to 12 hours, flipping after 30 minutes.

Preheat the oven to 375°F. Spray a baking sheet with nonstick cooking spray. Place the tofu on the baking sheet and bake for 20 minutes. Spray it with a little more cooking spray and flip the pieces. Spoon some marinade over each piece and bake another 10 minutes. If you like, place it under the broiler for about 3 more minutes for extra chewiness.

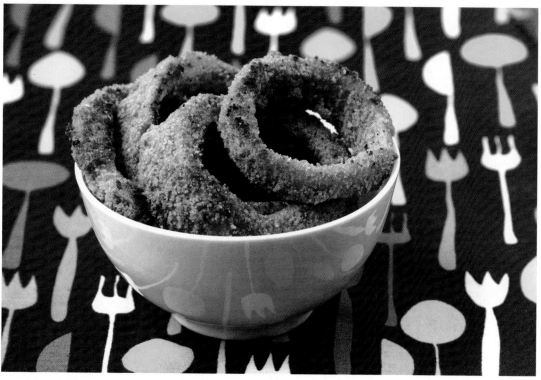

OMG Oven-Baked Onion Rings (page 59)

Spinach Lasagna with Roasted Cauliflower Ricotta & Spinach (page 179)

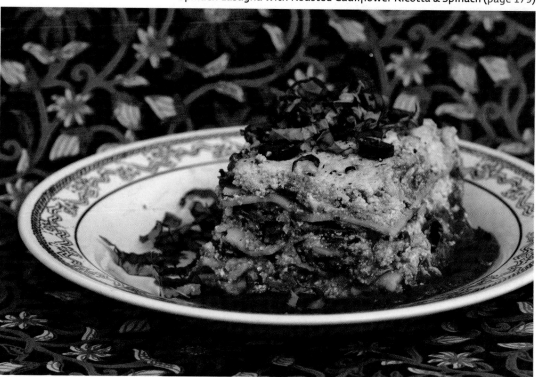

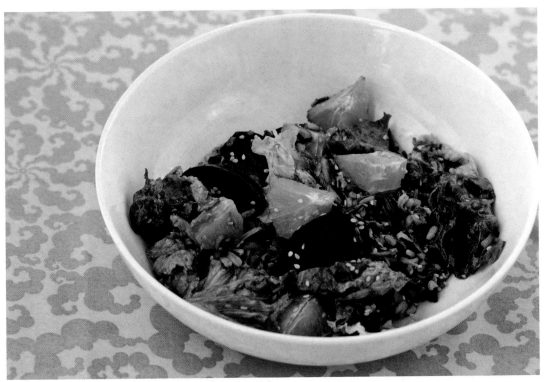

Wild Rice Salad with Oranges & Roasted Beets (page 39)

Sushi Roll Edamame Salad (page 20)

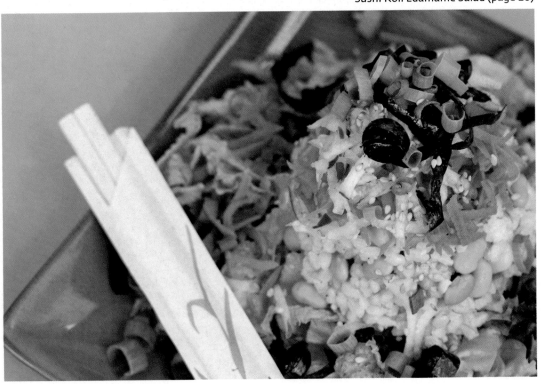

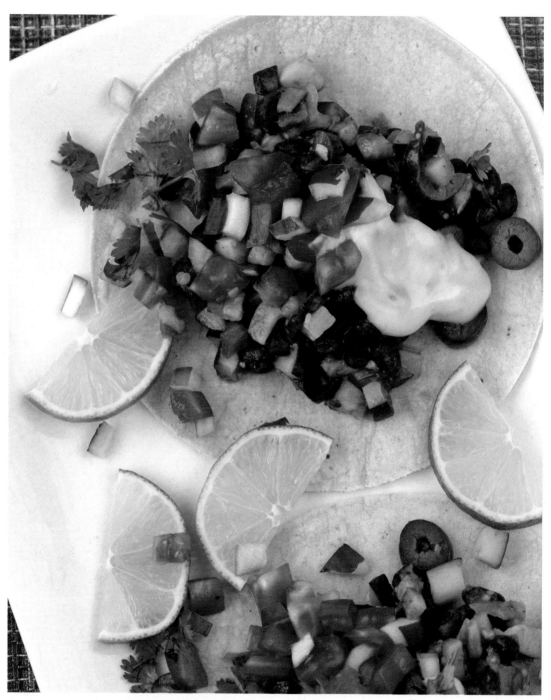

Black Bean, Zucchini, & Olive Tacos (page 131)

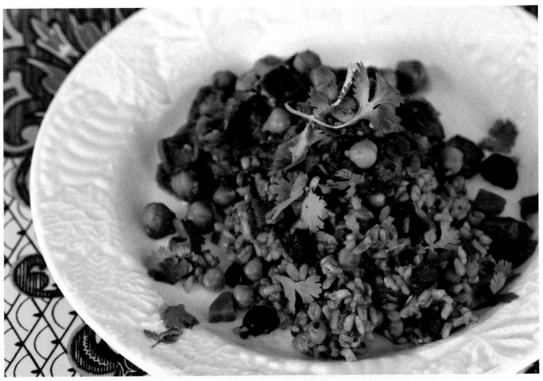

Eggplant-Chickpea Curry (page 230) and Cranberry-Cashew Biryani (page 67)

Quinoa, White Bean, & Kale Stew (page 245)

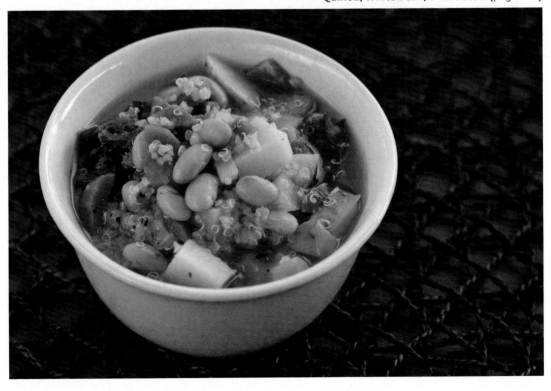

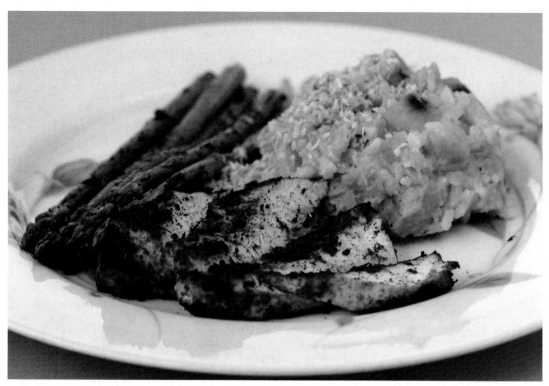

Broiled Blackened Tofu (page 147), Butternut Coconut Rice (page 80), and Jerk Asparagus (page 91)

Mushroom & Cannellini Paprikas (page 127) and Scarlet Barlety (page 69)

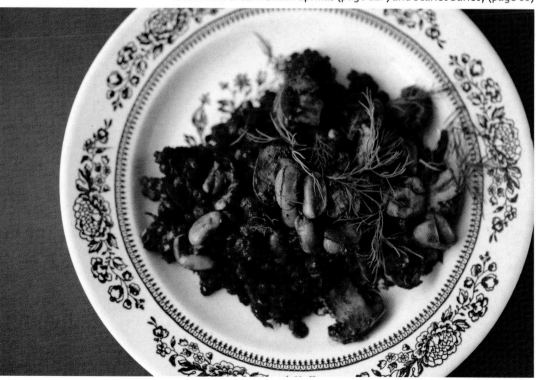

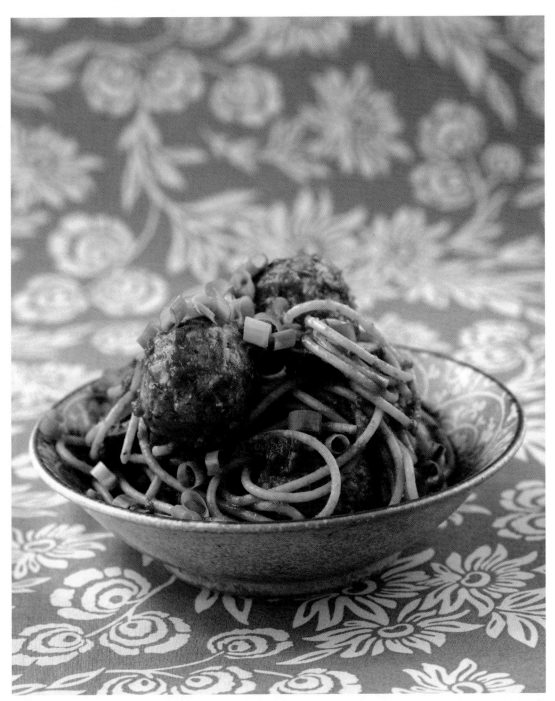

Cajun Beanballs & Spaghetti (page 190)

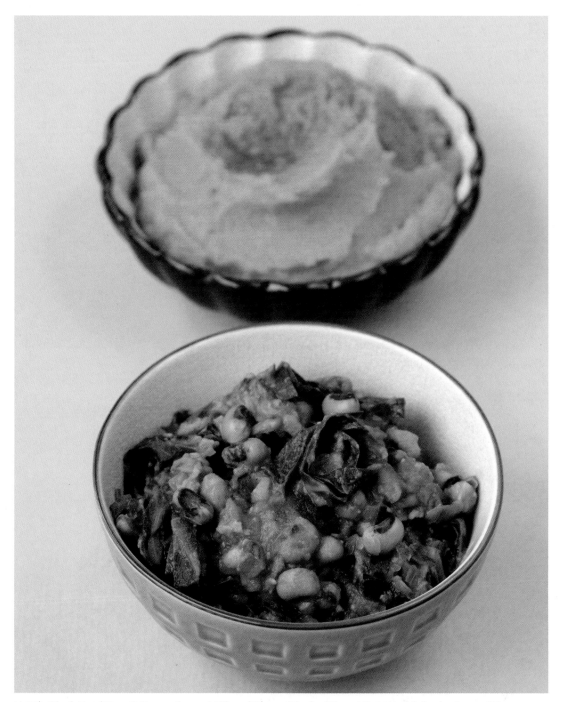

Hottie Black-Eyed Peas & Greens (page 119) and Ginger Mashed Sweet Potatoes & Apples (page 63)

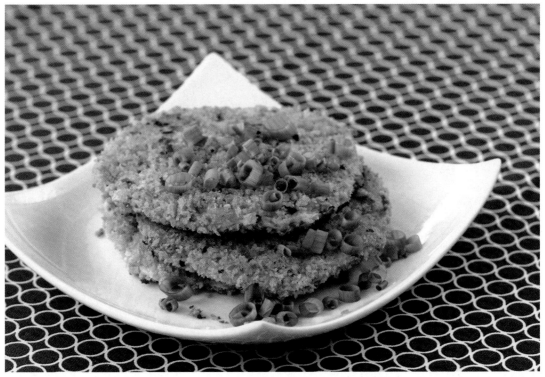

Scallion Potato Pancakes (page 61)

2nd Avenue Vegetable Korma (page 226)

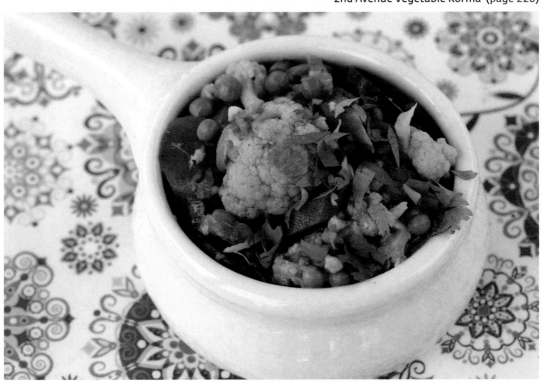

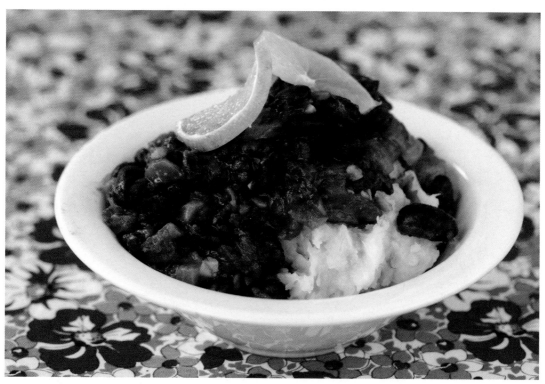

Mango BBQ Beans (page 133) and Mashed Yuca with Cilantro & Lime (page 57)

Veggie Potpie Stew (page 251) and Sweet Potato Drop Biscuits (page 253)

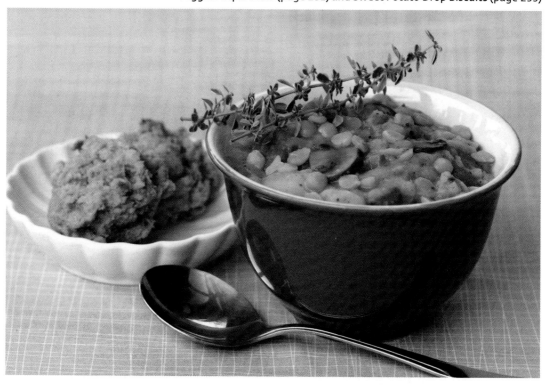

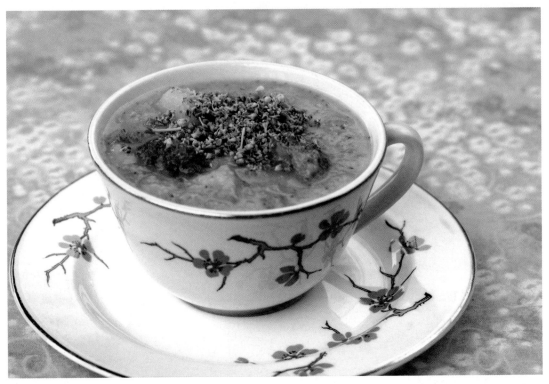

Bistro Broccoli Chowder (page 204)

Spinach Linguine with Edamame Pesto (page 174)

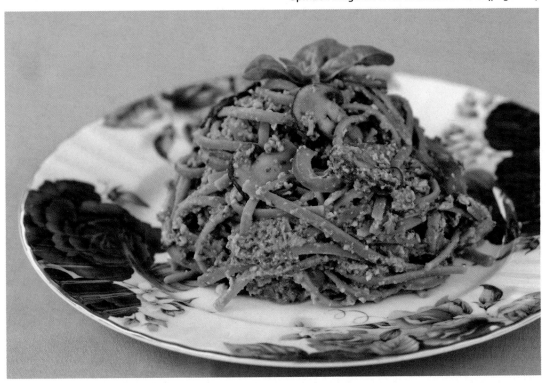

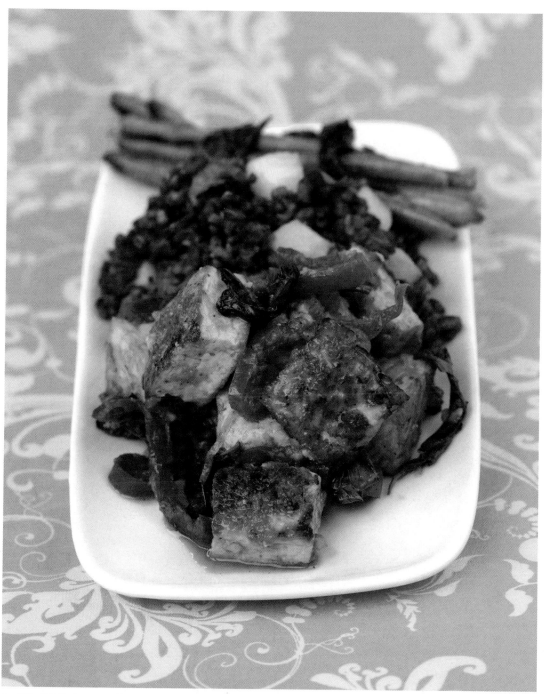

Red Thai Tofu (page 149), Bhutanese Pineapple Rice (page 72), and Green Beans with Thai Basil (page 98)

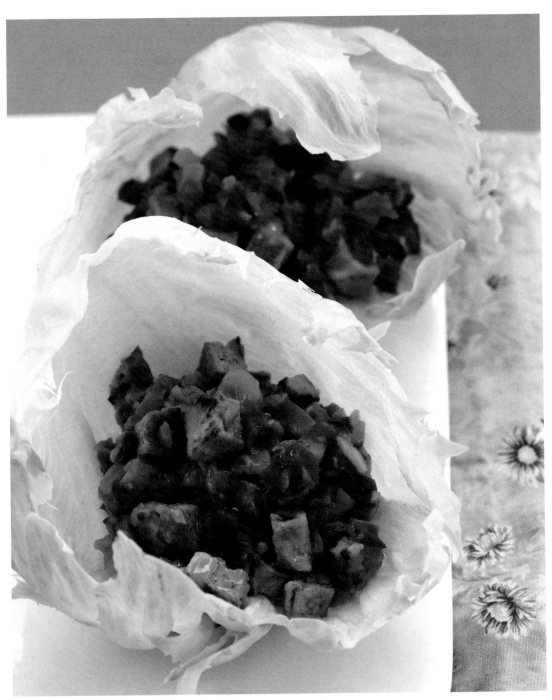

Lettuce Wraps with Hoison-Mustard Tofu (page 153)

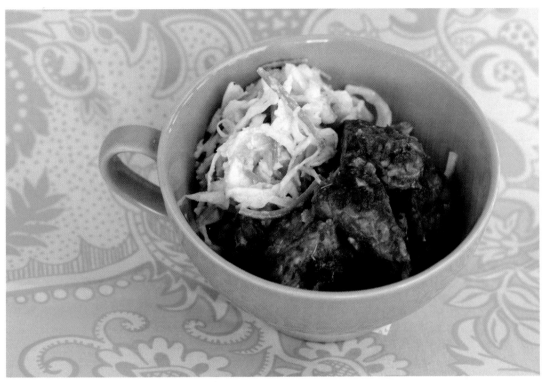

Buffalo Tempeh (page 161) with Cool Slaw (page 38)

Goddess Niçoise (page 25)

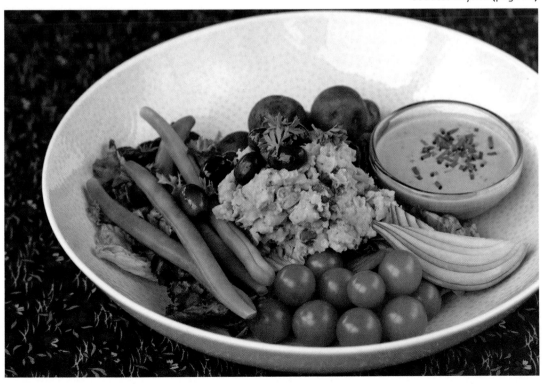

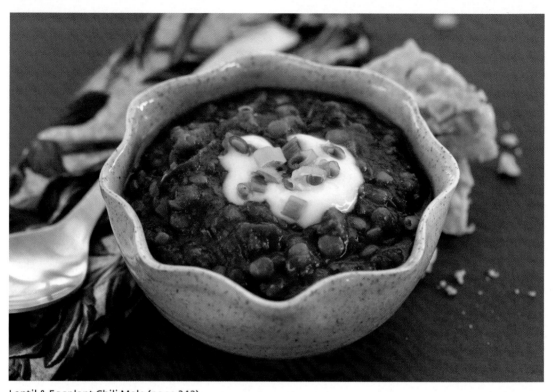

Lentil & Eggplant Chili Mole (page 242)

Tortilla Soup (page 208) and Fresh Corn & Scallion Corn Bread (page 244)

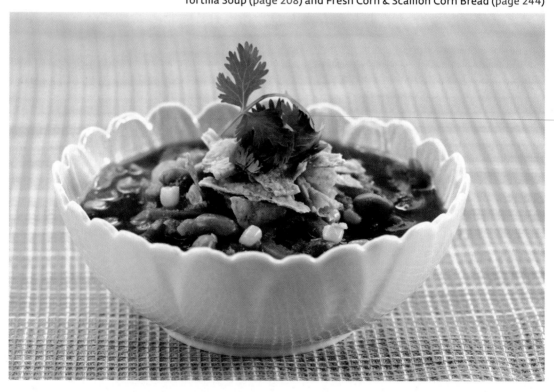

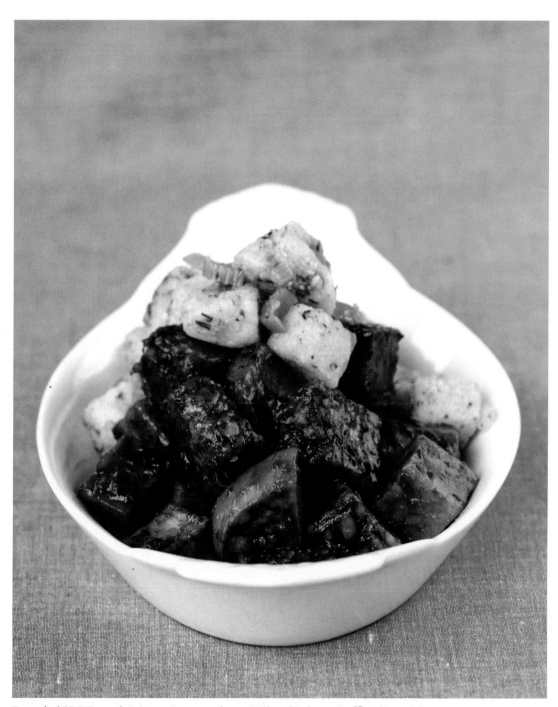

Tamarind BBQ Tempeh & Sweet Potatoes (page 159) and Polenta Stuffing (page 66)

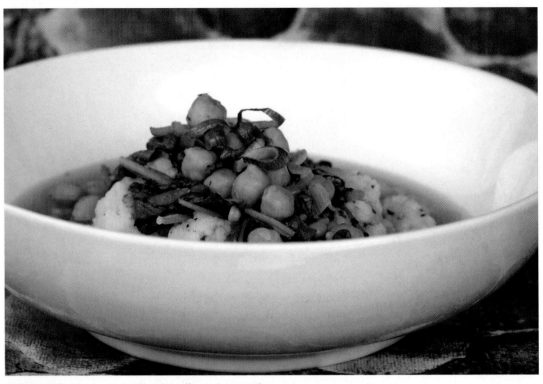

Chickpea Piccata (page 115) and Caulipots (page 54)

Caribbean Curried Black-Eyed Peas with Plantains (page 129)

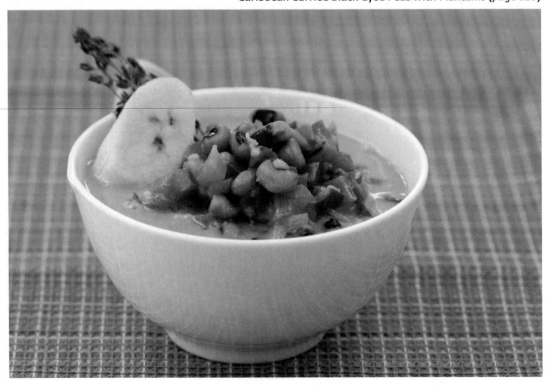

Broiled Blackened Tofu

SERVES 4 • ACTIVE TIME: 10 MINUTES • TOTAL TIME: 30 MINUTES

(CAN BE MADE GLUTEN FREE IF USING GF TAMARI)

Tofu is coated in Cajun spices and then cooked with high heat, so that it gets a nice crust. Booya, that is what blackening means! I've chosen to broil the tofu because this method doesn't require a whole lot of oil. Serve with **Butternut Coconut Rice** (page 80) and **Pineapple Collards** (page 93), or **Jerk Asparagus** (page 91)! If you want a lower-maintenance dinner, try it with the **Ginger Mashed Sweet Potato & Apples** (page 63).

SPICE BLEND:

2½ teaspoons sweet smoked paprika (see tip)
2 teaspoons ground cumin
1 teaspoon dried oregano
1 teaspoon dried thyme
1 teaspoon sugar
¼ teaspoon salt
¼ teaspoon cayenne
   Several pinches of freshly ground black pepper
3 cloves garlic, minced

EVERYTHING ELSE:

1 block tofu (about 14 ounces, pressed if you prefer), sliced into eighths
2 teaspoons olive oil
1 teaspoon soy sauce (use wheat-free tamari to keep it gluten free, if necessary)

On a dinner plate, mix together the spice blend and set aside.

Adjust the broiler (if necessary) so that the baking sheet will be around 6 inches away from the heat. Preheat the oven to broil. Spray a baking sheet with nonstick cooking spray. Poke each slice of tofu with a fork three or four times, to let the flavors seep in.

PER SERVING (¼ RECIPE):
Calories: 100
Calories from fat: 60
Total fat: 7 g
Saturated fat: 1 g
Trans fat: 0 g
Total carb: 5 g
Fiber: 2 g
Sugars: 2 g
Protein: 9 g
Cholesterol: 0 mg
Sodium: 240 mg
Vitamin A: 15%
Vitamin C: 4%
Calcium: 20%
Iron: 15%

TIP *You can press the tofu beforehand if you prefer a firmer bite (see page 143 for instructions). If you're pressed for time (no pun intended!), then don't worry about it; the tofu will be a bit more tender and juicy, which ain't exactly a bad thing.*

Drizzle the olive oil and soy sauce on the far side of the baking sheet, in a puddle. You'll be laying the tofu onto the sheet, so just make the "puddle" area off to one side. Dip each slice lightly into the sauce mixture, enough to lightly coat each side. Then dredge in the spice mixture, pressing firmly to make sure the spices will stick. Place the tofu on the baking sheet in a single layer. Spray the tops with a little cooking spray.

Place the tofu in the broiler and broil for about 12 minutes, flipping once about halfway through. Keep a close eye on it; broilers vary from oven to oven and you don't want your tofu to burn! The tofu is done when it looks dark and black in some spots. Thus the blackened! You can slice each piece into lengthwise strips, if you like. That makes for a nice presentation with the blackened crust and stark white interior. Serve ASAP.

TIP *If you're not sure if your smoked paprika is hot or sweet, then give it a taste test. Sweet paprika isn't exactly sweet, it's actually pleasantly bitter. The main point is, it isn't spicy. Hot paprika has a little kick to it. If it's hot paprika, just omit the cayenne and you should be all right.*

Red Thai Tofu

SERVES 4 • ACTIVE TIME: 20 MINUTES • TOTAL TIME: 30 MINUTES

(CAN BE MADE GLUTEN FREE IF USING GF TAMARI IN PLACE OF SOY SAUCE)

~~~~~~~~~~
PER SERVING
(¼ RECIPE):
Calories: 110
Calories from fat: 45
Total fat: 5 g
Saturated fat: 1 g
Trans fat: 0 g
Total carb: 10 g
Fiber: 2 g
Sugars: 4 g
Protein: 10 g
Cholesterol: 0 mg
Sodium: 780 mg
Vitamin A: 25%
Vitamin C: 70%
Calcium: 25%
Iron: 15%

Thai red curry paste is cheating a little bit, but so incredibly practical when you want Thai flavors such as lemongrass and galangal. This tofu comes together quickly, and because the marinade glazes the tofu, no long marinating time is required. Serve with **Bhutanese Pineapple Rice** (page 72) and **Green Beans with Thai Basil** (page 98).

- 1   block extra-firm tofu (about 14 ounces), cubed
- 1   red bell pepper, seeded and sliced thinly
- ½   cup sliced shallots
- 4   cloves garlic, minced
- 1   tablespoon minced fresh ginger
- 1   tablespoon Thai red curry paste
- ½   cup water
- 2   tablespoons soy sauce
- 1   tablespoon light agave nectar
- 15 leaves fresh Thai basil

Preheat a cast-iron or heavy-bottomed nonstick skillet over medium heat. Spray it with a little nonstick cooking spray. Add the tofu and cook for about 10 minutes, flipping it with a thin spatula once in a while, until it is browned on most sides. The thin spatula is important, because you should be able to slip it underneath the tofu and flip it easily, keeping the tofu intact. About midway through, drizzle with 2 teaspoons of the soy sauce and toss to coat.

Remove the tofu from the pan and set aside. Sauté the red pepper, shallots, garlic, and ginger in the oil, using a little cooking spray if needed. Cook for about 5 more minutes.

Meanwhile, in a small bowl, mix together the curry paste, water, remaining soy sauce, and agave. Add the tofu back to the pan along with the curry paste mixture. Cook for another 5 minutes. Add the Thai basil and toss to wilt. Serve!

Tofu Chimichurri

SERVES 4 • ACTIVE TIME: 20 MINUTES • TOTAL TIME: 1 HOUR 20 MINUTES

(CAN BE MADE GLUTEN FREE IF USING GF TAMARI IN PLACE OF SOY SAUCE)

Chimichurri is a marinade usually reserved for steak in Argentina, made from fresh herbs just plucked from your garden. Or, more likely, just plucked from the supermarket.

MARINADE:

¼ cup roughly chopped shallot
2 cloves garlic
1 cup loosely packed fresh cilantro
1 cup loosely packed fresh parsley
2 tablespoons soy sauce
¼ cup red wine vinegar
⅓ cup vegetable broth

TOFU:

1 block tofu (about 14 ounces), pressed

Chop the shallot and garlic in a food processor. Add the remaining ingredients and puree until relatively smooth.

Cut the tofu widthwise into eight equal pieces. If you like, slice those pieces corner to corner to form triangles. Marinate for at least an hour, flipping after 30 minutes.

Preheat a large skillet over medium-high heat. Spray the pan with a bit of nonstick cooking spray. Add the tofu slices and reserve the marinade. Cook the tofu for 10 minutes, flipping often, adding the marinade as you go. Add the remaining marinade and turn up the heat to high. Let the liquid boil and cook down for about 5 minutes. Serve!

Apple-Miso Tofu

SERVES 4 • ACTIVE TIME: 15 MINUTES • TOTAL TIME: 2 HOURS

**(CAN BE MADE GLUTEN FREE IF USING GF MISO AND GF TAMARI
IN PLACE OF SOY SAUCE)**

When you think "miso" you probably don't instantly think "apples," but they go incredibly well together. The very umami fermented flavor of miso is begging to be tempered by something sweet and fruity. Miso even has cidery undertones that make the pairing all the better. I hope I've made my case! Serve with brown basmati rice or **Scallion Potato Pancakes** (page 61) and **Orange-Scented Broccoli** (page 100). This is weeknight fare if you marinate the tofu early in the day and then just pop it in the oven when you're ready for dinner. If you press the tofu it will absorb more marinade, but it's not completely necessary.

MARINADE:

¼ cup water

5 tablespoons white miso

¼ cup mirin

1 tablespoon minced fresh ginger

3 cloves garlic, minced

2 tablespoons soy sauce

EVERYTHING ELSE:

1 teaspoon sesame oil

1 block extra-firm tofu (about 14 ounces)

1 pound red apples (2 large), peeled, cored, and cut into
½-inch-thick slices

Cooked rice, for serving

Arugula, chiffonaded (see tip, page 20) for garnish (optional)

Mix the marinade ingredients together in an 8 by 13-inch baking pan.

Cut the tofu widthwise into eight equal pieces. If you like, slice those pieces corner to corner to form triangles. Add the tofu and let marinate for about an hour, or up to 12 hours, flipping once to make sure everything gets coated.

Preheat the oven to 375°F. Add the apples to the pan; it's okay if they are not all submerged. Cover the pan tightly with tinfoil and bake for 30 minutes.

Remove the pan from the oven and remove the tinfoil. Bake for another 20 minutes. The tofu should be lightly browned and the apples should be nice and soft. Serve over rice and garnish with arugula, if desired.

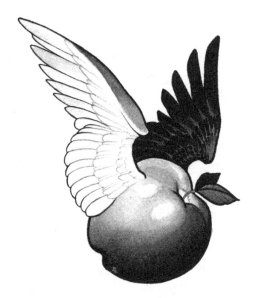

Lettuce Wraps with Hoisin-Mustard Tofu

SERVES 4 • ACTIVE TIME: 30 MINUTES • TOTAL TIME: 30 MINUTES

**(CAN BE MADE GLUTEN FREE IF USING GF HOISIN SAUCE AND
GF TAMARI IN PLACE OF SOY SAUCE)**

Iceberg lettuce gets a bad rap, but this is a really good wrap! Terrible puns aside, iceberg does provide the perfect pocket for this flavorful, Chinese-inspired glazed tofu. I love the contrast of cold and crisp with warm and sweet. The tofu is basically "fried" in a dry pan, coated with only a little bit of nonstick cooking spray. It gives the tofu a nice chewy exterior. You'll need a well-seasoned cast-iron pan for this, although a good-quality nonstick will work, too. Just avoid any cookware that has a tendency to stick. Serve with **Unfried Fried Rice** (page 70) and **Five-Spice Delicata Squash** (page 106), but remember to start those first since they take a while.

TOFU:

1 block extra-firm tofu (about 14 ounces), diced in ½-inch pieces

2 teaspoons soy sauce

SAUCE:

1 teaspoon sesame oil

1 red bell pepper, seeded and diced small

1 small onion, diced small

3 cloves garlic, minced

1 tablespoon minced fresh ginger

¼ teaspoon red pepper flakes (or ½ teaspoon if you want it spicier)

3 tablespoons mirin

2 tablespoons hoisin sauce

2 teaspoons prepared yellow mustard

TO SERVE:

About 12 iceberg lettuce leaves

**PER SERVING
(¼ RECIPE):**
Calories: 140
Calories from fat: 50
Total fat: 6 g
Saturated fat: 1 g
Trans fat: 0 g
Total carb: 16 g
Fiber: 2 g
Sugars: 8 g
Protein: 9 g
Cholesterol: 0 mg
Sodium: 440 mg
Vitamin A: 20%
Vitamin C: 70%
Calcium: 20%
Iron: 10%

Prepare the tofu: Preheat a cast-iron or heavy-bottomed nonstick skillet over medium heat. Spray it with a little nonstick cooking spray. Add the tofu and cook for about 10 minutes, flipping it with a thin spatula once in a while, until it is browned on most sides. The thin spatula is important, because you should be able to slip it underneath the tofu and flip it easily, keeping the tofu intact. About midway through, drizzle with the soy sauce and toss to coat.

Preheat a separate large pan over medium heat. Sauté the red pepper, onion, garlic, ginger, and red pepper flakes in the sesame oil, using a little cooking spray if needed. Cook for about 10 minutes. The veggies should be soft and browned. Add the mirin and let it cook out for about 3 minutes. Add the hoisin and mustard, and cook for about another minute.

Add the tofu to the sauce and toss to coat. Serve alongside lettuce leaves, to stuff like a taco.

> ∞ TIP This recipe calls for two pans because it's faster, but if you haven't got two large pans available, then just remove the tofu from the pan when done and then prepare the sauce right in that same pan. ∞

> ∞ TIP When prepping the lettuce leaves, some may rip, and that's okay. I found the easiest way to separate them without ripping is to cut off the bottom of the head, then carefully peel the leaves upward, instead of peeling from the tender tips of the leaves down. ∞

Chili-Lime-Rubbed Tofu

SERVES 4 • ACTIVE TIME: 10 MINUTES • TOTAL TIME: 30 MINUTES

(CAN BE MADE GLUTEN FREE IF USING GF TAMARI IN PLACE OF SOY SAUCE)

I f you don't have a hundred years (or an hour) to pump lots of flavor into your tofu via a marinade, then the next best thing is a super-flavorful coating. Enter "the rub." Rubbing tofu with assertive flavors, in this case chili powder and lime, is a great way to bring the noise to the dinner table. The noise being, "Mmmm . . ." This is great with **Pasta de los Angeles** (page 177).

1 block extra-firm tofu (about 14 ounces) sliced into
8 pieces widthwise
2 tablespoons mild chili powder
¼ teaspoon salt
¼ cup freshly squeezed lime juice (from about 2 limes)
1 teaspoon oil
1 teaspoon soy sauce
2 cloves garlic
Zest from 1 lime

Preheat the oven to 400°F. Poke each slice of tofu with a fork three or four times, to let the flavors seep in.

Mix together the chili powder and salt in a small ramekin and set aside.

Pour the lime juice, oil, and soy sauce into an 8 by 13-inch pan. Use a Microplane grater to grate in the garlic, and mix in the lime zest.

Toss each slice of tofu in the pan to coat with lime and stuff. Now rub each slice with a big pinch of the chili powder mixture, until well coated. Don't dredge the slices or they'll pick up too much coating. Arrange the tofu in the pan in a single layer.

Bake the tofu for 10 minutes on one side, flip it over, and bake for another 10 minutes. Serve!

**PER SERVING
(¼ RECIPE):**
Calories: 100
Calories from fat: 50
Total fat: 6 g
Saturated fat: 1 g
Trans fat: 0 g
Total carb: 6 g
Fiber: 2 g
Sugars: 1 g
Protein: 9 g
Cholesterol: 0 mg
Sodium: 280 mg
Vitamin A: 25%
Vitamin C: 15%
Calcium: 20%
Iron: 10%

TIP *Zest the lime before proceeding (because it's hard to zest a lime once it's been juiced.)*

Curried Scrambled Tofu with Wilted Arugula

SERVES 4 • ACTIVE TIME: 10 MINUTES • TOTAL TIME: 20 MINUTES

PER SERVING
(¼ RECIPE):
Calories: 100
Calories from fat: 50
Total fat: 5.5 g
Satured fat: 1 g
Trans fat: 0 g
Total carb: 7 g
Fiber: 2 g
Sugars: 2 g
Protein: 9 g
Cholesterol: 0 mg
Sodium: 450 mg
Vitamin A: 6%
Vitamin C: 10%
Calcium: 25%
Iron: 10%

Scrambled tofu is a quick, flavorful way to get your soy on, and I think it's one of the best recipes for tofu beginners. I have a bazillion different recipes for it, but this one is the simplest, most pantry-friendly, and in all my years of serving tofu, this one has been the most universally appealing. Wilting the arugula at the end gets you a nice splash of green without having to chop anything, so this can really be thrown together in no time flat.

    1 teaspoon olive oil
    1 medium-size red onion, diced finely
    3 cloves garlic, minced
    1 block extra-firm tofu (about 14 ounces)
2 to 3 teaspoons curry powder
    ½ teaspoon ground cumin
    1 tablespoons freshly squeezed lemon juice
    ¾ teaspoon salt
       A few pinches of freshly ground black pepper
    2 cups baby arugula

Preheat a large, heavy-bottomed pan over medium-high heat. Sauté the onion in the oil for about 4 minutes, until translucent. Add the garlic and sauté for 30 seconds or so. Crumble the tofu into bite-size pieces and add to the pan. Cook for about 10 minutes, stirring often, until the tofu has browned on some of the sides. Use a little nonstick cooking spray if needed.

Add the curry powder, cumin, salt, pepper, and a few splashes of water if it's too dry. Mix in the arugula. Cover and cook for 2 to 3 minutes, stirring occasionally, until the arugula is wilted.

Taste for spices and add another teaspoon of curry powder if needed; it will depend on the strength of your curry powder. Serve!

Red Wine & Kalamata Tempeh

SERVES 2 • ACTIVE TIME: 25 MINUTES • TOTAL TIME: 90 MINUTES

I've never been to Greece, but I imagine the vegan gods and goddesses would go crazy for this. Kalamata olives and red wine make for a succulent tempeh whose flavor just explodes in your mouth. Thin slices of tempeh ensure that the flavor is really absorbed. If you steam it for 5 minutes beforehand, it will absorb even more marinade and remove any bitter taste.

Serve with **Caulipots** (page 54) or a cup of whole wheat couscous and lots of steamed veggies, such as broccoli and zucchini. You heat up the marinade in the pan at the end, so it makes a great sauce to pour over everything.

8 ounces tempeh

MARINADE:
⅓ cup pitted kalamata olives
1 cup dry red wine
1 tablespoon balsamic vinegar
3 cloves garlic
2 teaspoons dried rosemary
1 teaspoon dried thyme
   Several pinches of freshly ground black pepper
   A pinch of salt
   A pinch of red pepper flakes

Prepare your steamer. Prepare the tempeh by slicing it widthwise into four equal pieces. Slice each of those pieces horizontally across the middle (like a clam) so that you have eight thin slices. Steam the tempeh for 5 minutes, if you like, and in the meantime prepare marinade.

Place all the marinade ingredients in a food processor or blender and pulse until the olives are pureed. They won't be completely smooth, but that's okay.

Pour the marinade into a mixing bowl or large zippered plastic bag.

PER SERVING
(½ RECIPE):
Calories: 370
Calories from fat: 80
Total fat: 8 g
Saturated fat: 1 g
Trans fat: 0 g
Total carb: 36 g
Fiber: 10 g
Sugars: 2 g
Protein: 18 g
Cholesterol: 0 mg
Sodium: 380 mg
Vitamin A: 50%
Vitamin C: 4%
Calcium: 10%
Iron: 6%

Add the tempeh and let marinate for at least an hour or up to overnight, flipping once if needed to make sure the flavor absorbs evenly.

Preheat a large, heavy-bottomed skillet (preferably cast-iron) over medium heat. Spray it with nonstick cooking spray, then add the tempeh in a single layer.

Cook for 15 minutes, flipping every few minutes and adding marinade as needed to keep the tempeh from getting dry. In the last minute or so, add the remainder of the marinade and turn up the heat to bring to a boil. Let boil for about 3 minutes.

Serve over Caulipots and veggies, and make sure to pour the remaining sauce over everything, for lots of flavor.

❧ INGREDIENT SCAVENGER HUNT

Kalamata olives are named for a city where they originate, in Greece, but they are sold in many supermarkets these days. They are a dark maroon and have a meaty texture and sultry taste. Although they're commonly sold in jars, fresher is better. Fancy stores like Whole Foods Market often have an olive bar, where you can sneak a taste before packing them up (don't tell them I sent you.) Or if you have a Mediterranean market nearby, even better! In NYC, these markets are often called "International" or "Gourmet" or sometimes "International Gourmet," for good measure. ✎

Tamarind BBQ Tempeh & Sweet Potatoes

SERVES 4 • ACTIVE TIME: 15 MINUTES • TOTAL TIME: 70 MINUTES

(CAN BE MADE GLUTEN FREE IF USING GF TAMARI IN PLACE OF SOY SAUCE)

Tart tamarind is often a secret ingredient in BBQ sauces, but I love it as an in-your-face, not-so-secret ingredient. I also love that this dish comes all together in one pan, with minimal prep. The sauce glazes the tempeh and sweet potatoes and creates the perfect mingling of sweet, tangy, savory, and smoky. The longer you marinate, the more flavor will permeate the tempeh.

You can even assemble this the night before or the morning of, store in the fridge, and pop into the oven when you're ready to go. If you're going to skip the marinating phase, then remember to preheat the oven while you're prepping the veggies. Serve with **Polenta Stuffing** (page 66) and **Shaved Brussels Sprouts** (page 92) for a Thanksgiving dinner that will have your hot pants thanking you. You can also just serve with some rice and a green.

~~~~~~~~~~~
PER SERVING
(¼ RECIPE):
Calories: 380
Calories from fat: 45
Total fat: 5 g
Saturated fat: 0.5 g
Trans fat: 0 g
Fiber: 13 g
Protein: 17 g
Cholesterol: 0 mg
Sodium: 780 mg
Vitamin A: 530%
Vitamin C: 10%
Calcium: 15%
Iron: 10%

SAUCE:

- 4 cloves garlic, minced
- 1 tablespoon minced fresh ginger
- ¾ cup vegetable broth
- 2 teaspoons arrowroot dissolved in ¼ cup water
- 2 tablespoons tomato paste
- 1 tablespoon tamarind concentrate
- 3 tablespoons agave or maple syrup
- 2 tablespoons soy sauce
- 1 teaspoon olive oil
- 1 teaspoon liquid smoke
- ⅛ teaspoon cayenne (optional)

1½ pounds sweet potatoes, peeled and sliced in ¾-inch chunks

12 ounces tempeh, cut into ¾-inch cubes

Spray a 9 by 13-inch casserole pan with nonstick cooking spray. If using glass (which I don't recommend! But I can't stop you!), then line the bottom with parchment paper to prevent sticking.

In a medium-size mixing bowl, whisk together all the sauce ingredients. Make sure to get the tamarind dissolved.

Place the sweet potatoes and tempeh in the prepared pan. Pour the sauce over them and use your hands to coat well. You can bake immediately or let marinate for at least an hour to get more flavor into the tempeh.

When ready to bake, preheat the oven to 400°F. Cover the pan with tinfoil and bake for about 25 minutes. Remove from the oven and toss out the tinfoil. Flip the tempeh and sweet potatoes, making sure to scrape the bottom with a spatula in case anything is sticking. Bake for another half hour, flipping everything once. The sweet potatoes should be tender but not mushy, and the sauce should be thickened and coating everything. Serve!

Buffalo Tempeh

SERVES 4 • ACTIVE TIME: 15 MINUTES • TOTAL TIME: 30 MINUTES

(CAN BE MADE GLUTEN FREE IF USING GF HOT SAUCE)

ot sauce lovers only! When you're craving something spicy, saucy, and greasy, this tempeh does the trick. The thing is, they aren't actually greasy or fatty, they only look like they are. There's no oil in the marinade, and don't be suspicious that it contains only four ingredients; plenty of garlic and oregano will make you crave these winglike tempeh wedges even when you're not watching the big game. I love to mix this sauce with **Mac & Trees** (page 184), so pour some **Easy Breezy Cheezy Sauce** (page 173) over your macaroni and then top it with Buffalo Tempeh. Or, try Buffalo Tempeh with **Cool Slaw** (page 38). Anything creamy and cooling will be great with this recipe.

8 ounces tempeh, cut into wedges (see below)

MARINADE:

½ cup vegetable broth

½ cup cayenne hot sauce

6 cloves garlic, minced

2 teaspoons dried oregano

To create wedges, slice the tempeh in half across the waist. Slice the resulting square in half. You'll have four rectangles. Slice each of those rectangles corner to corner. The resulting triangular wedges are great for baking, grilling, or sautéing.

Prepare your steaming apparatus. Steam the tempeh for 5 minutes; this will loosen the tempeh up and get it ready to absorb the marinade flavors.

Mix together the marinade ingredients in a medium-size mixing bowl. When the tempeh is done steaming, immediately transfer it to the marinade. Let it marinate for at least 10 minutes, up to an hour.

PER SERVING
(¼ RECIPE):
Calories: 130
Calories from fat: 20
Total fat: 2.5 g
Saturated fat: 0 g
Trans fat: 0 g
Total carb: 18 g
Fiber: 5 g
Sugars: 1 g
Protein: 9 g
Cholesterol: 0 mg
Sodium: 290 mg
Vitamin A: 30%
Vitamin C: 4%
Calcium: 6%
Iron: 2%

Preheat a large skillet over medium-high heat. Spray the pan with a bit of nonstick cooking spray. Add the tempeh slices and reserve the marinade. Cook the tempeh for 10 minutes, flipping it often, until it has browned a bit. Add the remaining sauce and turn up the heat to high. Let the liquid boil and cook down for about 5 minutes. That's it!

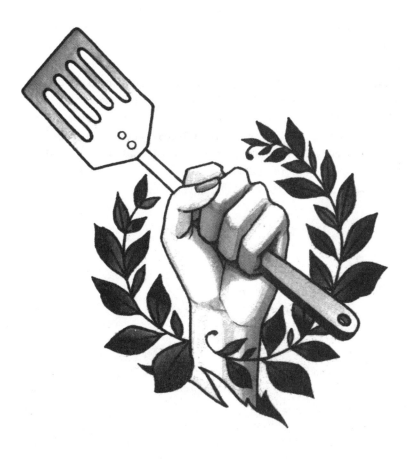

CHAPTER 6

Talk Pasta to Me (& Noodles!)

OH, THOSE CARB-FEARING '90S. THEY HAD EVERYONE RUN FOR the hills the moment a forkful of pasta was spotted. Look at them all, slurping up those long strands of fettuccine (a.k.a. pure evil), dripping with sauce, washing it down with wine . . . surely if you're enjoying life, there has got to be a price to pay! And so they took to their ThighMasters, cursing the carb eaters and weeping into their Atkins bars.

But guess what? Pasta is good for you! From Italian favorites such as lasagna, macaroni, and linguine to Japanese staples such as soba and udon, this chapter does not discriminate. We embrace each and every noodle—spirals, ridges, curves, and all. The key with pasta is limiting refined carbs and upping the fiber, and there are a variety of pastas that make it easy to do so.

You don't need to employ outdated weight-loss techniques to make pasta a meal you can enjoy. No need to use a tiny bowl to make the meal look larger, or to put the fork down between every bite. In fact, use the biggest bowl you've got and fill that bowl—but with veggies, sauce, and beans. A 2-ounce (uncooked) serving of pasta may look skimpy on its own but really (honestly! truly!) is enough, once you've bulked it up. You'll learn lots of cooking tech-

What is complex about a carbohydrate?

At its most basic, a carbohydrate is fuel for our body. All carbs end up as glucose, but in nutrition, as in life (or on road trips to see your best friend's cousin's band in faraway Canadian cities), sometimes the journey is more important than the destination. Complex carbohydrates take longer for our body to digest, keep us full longer, and don't cause our blood sugar to spike. Unlike simple carbohydrates (such as sugar and white bread), complex carbohydrates have fiber and other nutrients that are important to maintain weight and to keep us healthy.

niques from this chapter, but let's start with a few rules of thumb.

I haven't met a veggie that doesn't do well sautéed with a lot of garlic and some freshly ground black pepper. Throw some pasta into the mix and you've got yourself a meal. Many veggies release lots of tasty juices when cooking, but add some veggie broth to help it along. Check out the **Pasta con Broccoli** recipe (page 169) for a base, but also check out the veggie chapter. Recipes like **Sautéed Escarole** (page 107), **Garlicky Mushrooms & Kale** (page 89), and **Shaved Brussels Sprouts** (page 92) are dying to be tossed with some pasta. And don't be scared of using pasta in nontraditional (read: not Italian) ways. Those **Mushroom Tibs** (page 95) or **Curried Cabbage and Peas** (page 111) would make great pasta dishes. Also, check out the veggie steaming chapter and add your favorites to pasta, then smother in sauces. Maybe you have some veggie favorites that you can adapt into pasta dishes.

> ∾ TIP _It's fairly rare with dried varieties, but once in a while, egg or dairy products sneak their way into your pasta's ingredients list. It never hurts to check the ingredients, especially with the ease of bolded allergy information that most packaging has these days._ ∾

A handful of beans goes a long way in pastas. Some of my favorites to use are kidney, cannellini, my beloved chickpea, and navy or great northern beans. But don't just toss the beans in at the end, add them to the veggies in the pan and let them cook for a few minutes so that they absorb some flavor. Also, check out the **Miso Udon Stir-fry with Greens & Beans** (page 95) and **Pasta de los Angeles** (page 111) for unorthodox use of beans in pasta. You can also use some of the bean recipes as sauce bases for pasta. The **Chickpea Piccata** (page 115) and **Mushroom-Cannellini Paprikas** (page 127), are both good contenders.

And no need to skimp on the sauce! Use fresh tomato or marinara sauces, broth-based garlicky sauces, or any of the sauces in this chapter and pour them on. You might even like some of the dressings in this section as pasta sauces; you never know.

Bon appétit!

∾ PERFECT PASTA TOOL CHECKLIST ∾

- 4-quart pot
- Pasta spoon (that's a large spoon with rounded prongs, making it easy to stir and serve the pasta)
- Big colander

And just a last note about time management: To get your pasta dishes on the table in under 30 minutes, remember to start boiling the water before you do anything else. In the 10 minutes it takes to boil the water, you can probably get all your prepping done and even have some onions and veggies sautéing away.

The Pocket Pasta Guide

Not all pastas are created equal! Store this info in your brain for the next time you are standing dumbfounded in the pasta aisle.

SEMOLINA (A.K.A. REGULAR OLD PASTA)

Semolina pasta, made from durum wheat, may be somewhat nutritionally inferior to whole wheat, but it's not without some good nutrition. If white pasta is your thing, well, go for it; it certainly won't kill you. It has about 2 grams of fiber per 2-ounce serving and it is enriched with iron and B vitamins. When you load it up with nutrient-dense, fiber-rich vegetables, enriched pasta can be a healthy vehicle for a plant-based meal.

WHOLE WHEAT PASTA

Whole wheat pasta is much more than starch. The complex carbohydrates and 5 grams of fiber keep you feeling full and have a lower glycemic index than does enriched pasta, meaning it won't spike your blood sugar. A 2-ounce serving has a whopping 8 grams of protein and naturally occurring iron and B vitamins that are lost when whole grains are refined. It's also a good source of magnesium, which is a cofactor for hundreds of enzymes, including how insulin and glucose are used by the body.

New whole wheat brands are popping up all the time, so definitely keep an open mind (and an open shopping cart) and give a few different kinds a shot. My favorite brand right now is Bionaturae: It not only tastes the closest to good old semolina pasta, but it has lots of organic varieties, so you can eat your fusilli and have a planet, too. I prefer to use whole wheat pasta when I'm working with long, skinny varieties, such as spaghetti and linguine. Oh, and be on the lookout for deceptive packaging. Sometimes pasta labels will say something like, "Wheat pasta" or "Contains whole wheat." Read the ingredients list and make sure that "whole wheat" is the main ingredient. "Wheat flour" or "semolina wheat flour" doesn't mean it's made from actual whole wheat.

BROWN RICE PASTA (GLUTEN-FREE)

Brown rice pasta is my favorite gluten-free option. In fact, I prefer the taste and texture to that of whole wheat pasta. I go brown rice pasta when I'm making dishes that require small shapes, such as macaroni or little shells.

Brown rice pasta can be lower in protein and fiber than the other whole-grain pastas, but it's full of complex carbohydrates and is completely fat free. If you're avoiding gluten, then this pasta is certainly a chef's best friend.

QUINOA PASTA (GLUTEN-FREE)

Quinoa pasta is just what it sounds like—pasta made from ground quinoa. So it has a lot of the same nutritional benefits of quinoa, including essential amino acids, which are the building blocks of protein.

It's also got plenty of iron and fiber. The texture is smooth and chewy, pretty close to that of semolina pasta, but it has a more pronounced healthy taste. If that sort of thing bugs you, then try it with a strongly flavored sauce, as in the **Tempeh Helper** (page 171).

CORN PASTA (GLUTEN-FREE)

I don't call for corn pasta specifically in any of my recipes, but it's definitely worth a mention. Corn pasta usually has two very simple ingredients, which is a great sign when you're aiming to eat a whole-foods diet. And it is very high in fiber, upward of 6 grams per serving, but be sure to read the nutrition label of the brand you use.

SPINACH OR OTHER FLAVORED PASTAS

These are usually white pastas that have powdered vegetables that give them color, but some brands just have color. Be sure to read the nutrient label to make sure that the spinach in your pasta is real spinach. Nutritionally speaking, such blends as spinach or tomato don't bring too much to the party, but they do look pretty and taste great.

Pasta Primer

Is there anything worse than a clump of pasta, or noodles that are undercooked in some places and overcooked in others? No, not really. Dick Cheney probably cooks his pasta like that, that's how awful it is. Don't be like Dick Cheney, cook your pasta properly!

1. First things first, and that first thing is the vehicle you're going to use to cook. For 8 ounces of dry pasta, I use a 4-quart, heavy-bottomed, stainless-steel pot with a long handle. The long handle really helps for when it comes time to drain. The heavy bottom (I love saying "heavy bottom") keeps things evenly heated.

2. Fill the pot three-quarters full with water; you want plenty of room for your pasta to float around in to prevent it from sticking together.

3. Salt the water. Like, *really* salt it, with about a tablespoon of salt. Salt flavors the pasta, keeping it from tasting bland.

4. Bring the water to a full, rolling boil before adding the pasta. This is super important for getting pasta evenly cooked and to keep it from clumping together. Once the pasta is added, bring it back up to a full boil and stir frequently with a pasta spoon to keep it from sticking together.

5. Taste the pasta to see if it's done. There's that theory that if you throw it at the wall and it sticks it's done, and I don't know how accurate that is. What I do know is that it will make a mess of your wall. Just taste it and save your walls the trouble.

6. If the recipe calls for draining, have a big colander at the ready. But don't leave the cooked pasta sitting around for too long, or it will stick together.

Fusilli Roasted Veggie Primavera

SERVES 4 • ACTIVE TIME: 20 MINUTES • TOTAL TIME: 50 MINUTES

(CAN BE MADE GLUTEN FREE IF USING GF FUSILLI)

Let's start this pasta chapter off fresh and simple. Primavera means "early spring," and spring means veggies! Or something like that. Roasting coaxes so much flavor out of summer's early harvest veggies, so very little herbs and spices are needed. Cherry tomatoes burst just a bit while roasting, creating just enough saucy juice to make this dish work. A splash of balsamic vinegar at the end brings everything together. I love the fun shape of fusilli here and how its curves soak up flavor.

½ pound whole wheat fusilli
1 pound zucchini, sliced ¼ inch thick
1 pound yellow squash, sliced ¼ inch thick
½ pound asparagus, coarse ends discarded, cut into 1-inch pieces
1 red bell pepper, seeded and sliced ¼ inch thick
1 small red onion, cut into ¼-inch-thick half-moons
1½ cups cherry tomatoes
6 cloves garlic, minced
2 teaspoons dried oregano
2 teaspoons dried thyme
1 tablespoon olive oil
1 teaspoon salt
Freshly ground black pepper
2 tablespoons balsamic vinegar
Fresh basil, for garnish (optional)

Preheat the oven to 450°F. Line two large baking sheets with parchment paper and mist with nonstick cooking spray.

PER SERVING (¼ RECIPE):
Calories: 320
Calories from fat: 45
Total fat: 5
Saturated fat: 1 g
Trans fat: 0 g
Fiber: 11 g
Protein: 14 g
Cholesterol: 0 mg
Sodium: 610 mg
Vitamin A: 45%
Vitamin C: 150%
Calcium: 10%
Iron: 30%

Place all the veggies in a large mixing bowl along with oregano and thyme. Drizzle with olive oil and sprinkle with salt and pepper. Use your hands to toss, making sure all the veggies are coated. Place the veggies in a single layer on both pans. Bake for 15 minutes on separate racks, remove them from the oven, and flip the veggies. You don't have to be too precise about this; just take a minute to do your best. Now is also a good time to boil water for the pasta. Place the veggies back in the oven, putting the pan that was on the top rack on the bottom and vice versa. Bake for 15 more minutes, or until tender. The asparagus tips should be frizzled, the zuke should be tender, and the tomatoes should be bursting. While the veggies are finishing their roast, cook the pasta according to the package directions, drain in a colander, and set aside.

Once the veggies are done, transfer them back to the big mixing bowl. This should be easy to do by just lifting the parchment and sliding them in. Toss with the balsamic vinegar.

Add the fusilli and toss to coat. Taste for salt and pepper and serve, topping with fresh basil if desired.

> **∾ BULK IT UP** Chickpeas would be great here. Just place 1½ cups on a baking sheet in the last 5 minutes of cooking. Or you can top with **Baked Tofu** (page 144) or **Red Wine & Kalamata Tempeh** (page 157). ∾

Pasta con Broccoli

SERVES 4 • ACTIVE TIME: 20 MINUTES • TOTAL TIME: 30 MINUTES

(CAN BE MADE GLUTEN FREE IF USING GF LINGUINE)

O r maybe I should call this Broccoli con Pasta? Meat eaters are fond of saying things like, "You don't crave broccoli the way I crave steak!" But I think the ferocity with which I devour a stalk of broccoli deserves its own two-part special on Animal Planet. I make this dish for my sister who likes very simple food: plain bagels and pretzels without salt (weirdo). She almost always orders Pasta con Broccoli when we go to Italian restaurants, while everyone else fills up on big sloppy dishes covered in red sauce. I used to raise my eyebrows at her, but somehow always end up taking a bite that turns into ten bites until she gets mad at me. What I'm saying is simple food can be the best kind, and these days a big old bowl of Pasta con Broccoli is perfect comfort food.

I make mine just a bit spicy with crushed red pepper and ground black pepper, but adjust as you see fit. Traditionally the dish is drowning in olive oil; here, we use just a bit for sautéing the garlic and then opt for veggie broth and white wine for a light sauce. And speaking of the garlic, there is a ton of it in here and I prep it two ways to get the biggest, most garlicky bang—half is minced and half is sliced.

½	pound whole wheat linguine
2	teaspoons olive oil
¼	cup thinly sliced garlic
3	cloves garlic, minced
½	teaspoon red pepper flakes
1	teaspoon dried thyme
1	cup vegetable broth
½	cup dry white wine
½	teaspoon salt
4	cups broccoli, tops cut into small florets, stalks sliced thinly
2	teaspoons balsamic vinegar
	Several pinches of freshly ground black pepper

**PER SERVING
(¼ RECIPE):**
Calories: 300
Calories from fat: 30
Total fat: 3.5 g
Saturated fat: 0.5 g
Trans fat: 0 g
Total carb: 54 g
Fiber: 7 g
Sugars: 5 g
Protein: 12 g
Cholesterol: 0 mg
Sodium: 470 mg
Vitamin A: 10%
Vitamin C: 140%
Calcium: 10%
Iron: 15%

Bring a large pot of salted water to a boil and prep all your ingredients while the water boils, because this dish comes together in no time. Once boiling, add the pasta and cook per the package directions, usually for about 10 minutes.

Preheat a large nonstick skillet over medium heat. Sauté the garlic, red pepper flakes, and thyme in the oil for about a minute, being careful not to burn them. Stir in the vegetable broth, wine, and salt. Add the broccoli, turn up the heat to bring it to a simmer, and cover the pan. Cook for 8 to 13 minutes, depending on how soft or firm you like your broccoli, stirring occasionally.

When the pasta is done cooking, drain and add it to the pan, using a pasta spoon to toss it around for about 3 more minutes, making sure to get everything coated. Mix in the balsamic vinegar. Serve with generous doses of black pepper. There is usually a lot of garlic left in the pan, so be sure to spoon that over your bowls of pasta.

> ✆ BULK IT UP *If you need some protein with your meal, try either* **Basic Baked Tofu (or Tempeh)** *(page 144). If you aren't feeling like soy at the moment, add a can of drained chickpeas or white beans when you add the pasta to the pan.* ✆

> ✆ TIP *To get some healthy fats and a whole lotta flavor into the dish, add a tablespoon of toasted pine nuts to each serving. It's also nice to top with a tablespoon of nutritional yeast, if you swing that way.* ✆

> ✆ NUTRITION TIP *Broccoli comes bundled as a good source of calcium, iron, and B vitamins, and a very good source of fiber, vitamin A, vitamin C, vitamin K, and folate. The large amount of vitamin C (found in the florets; the darker the better) significantly improves your body's absorption of the iron in the broccoli and the whole wheat pasta. Most of the nutrients are found in the florets, but the stem is full of healthy insoluble fiber, plus adds great texture to this dish.* ✆

Tempeh Helper

SERVES 4 • ACTIVE TIME: 20 MINUTES • TOTAL TIME: 30 MINUTES

This recipe is all about my childhood. My mom was raising three kids and working two jobs, so most of the action on our stove top came from a box. Still, it was fun to help her put away groceries, open cartons, and put together dinner. And because chopping veggies would take 15 minutes of time and energy she didn't have, we'd dump in the box of Hamburger Helper and that was that.

Now, of course, I know better. That box is wasteful and full of nasty ingredients, and of course, meat is murder. But I still get a taste for the Helper; the comforting aroma, the meaty bites, the chewy pasta that maybe gets a little burned on the bottom of the pan. And oh yeah, that velvety processed cheese product topping!

This version is quick, tasty, healthier, and still comes together in one pot. Tempeh has a succulent bite, and although I usually cringe at the idea of granulated garlic and onion flakes, that's what really gives this authenticity. Tiny quinoa shells are quick cooking thanks to their diminutive size, and are a nice healthy alternative to semolina pasta, but you can use whatever kind you like. You also might like that there is no cutting.

PER SERVING
(¼ RECIPE):
Calories: 310
Calories from fat: 45
Total fat: 5 g
Saturated fat: 1 g
Trans fat: 0 g
Total carb: 52 g
Fiber: 7 g
Sugars: 3 g
Protein: 16 g
Cholesterol: 0 mg
Sodium: 210 mg
Vitamin A: 35%
Vitamin C: 4%
Calcium: 8%
Iron: 15%

1   recipe **Easy Breezy Cheezy Sauce** (recipe follows)
1   teaspoon olive oil
8   ounces tempeh
3   cups water
6   ounces small shell pasta, or about a cup (I use quinoa pasta)
    A handful of frozen peas, about ¼ cup

SEASONING MIX:
2   teaspoons onion flakes
1   teaspoon garlic
1   teaspoon dried thyme
1   teaspoon dried oregano
1   teaspoon mild chili powder

⅛ teaspoon freshly ground black pepper
2 tablespoon broth powder (I used Frontier chicken-style broth)
2 teaspoons arrowroot or cornstarch
Salt

Preheat a large skillet over medium heat. Have a lid at the ready because you'll need to cover it at some point.

Drizzle the oil in the pan and spray with nonstick cooking spray. Tear the tempeh into bite-size pieces, adding them to the pan. Sauté for about 5 minutes, until the tempeh is lightly browned. Use cooking spray as needed. In the meantime, mix the seasonings together in a mixing bowl.

Add a few tablespoons of water to the tempeh to deglaze the pan. Add the 3 cups of water and the seasoning mixture, giving a good stir to get it all mixed in. Add the pasta and cover. Bring up the heat to a boil. Once the water is boiling, you can lower the heat to a simmer. Cook for about 10 minutes, stirring once. Remove the lid, add the peas, and cook until the sauce is reduced and thickened to your liking, usually about 3 minutes. Taste for salt and serve.

∽ TIP *If you'd like to quadruple this mix to have on hand, keep it refrigerated and just scoop out a heaping ¼ cup full whenever you get the hankering.* ∽

∽ BULK IT UP *There is plenty of sauce to go around here, so why not steam a bunch of broccoli to go along with everything?* ∽

∽ TIP *For maximum time management, begin the cheezy sauce first, and let it thicken while you prepare everything else. It will still come out in 30 minutes!* ∽

Easy Breezy Cheezy Sauce

MAKES 2 CUPS, OR EIGHT ¼-CUP SERVINGS • ACTIVE TIME: 10 MINUTES •
TOTAL TIME: 20 MINUTES

Nutritional yeast–based "cheese" sauces are a vegan tradition.
Recipes like this have been appearing in vegan cookbooks since
the dawn of time (or at least the seventies). The upside, they taste like
cheese! Or at least like junk food–type cheese, but it isn't junk food at all.
The downside, they are often loaded with fat! I mean loaded. One of the
most famous recipes for vegan cheese sauce calls for ½ cup of margarine. This is my waaaay slimmed-down version, which has no added fat
at all. It's still a thick and luscious bright orange cheezy sauce, perfect
for pastas and veggies.

- ¾ cup nutritional yeast
- ¼ cup all-purpose flour
- 2 teaspoons granulated garlic
- 2 teaspoons onion flakes
- ¼ teaspoon salt, or to taste
- ⅛ teaspoon ground turmeric
- 2 tablespoons broth powder (I used Frontier chicken-style broth)
- 2 cups water
- 1 teaspoon prepared yellow mustard

Place the nutritional yeast, flour, garlic, onion flakes, salt, turmeric, and
broth powder in a bowl and mix together. Add the water and use a fork
to mix and beat out any big lumps. Once relatively smooth, pour into a
2-quart saucepot. Turn up the heat to medium-high and cook, stirring
often, for about 5 minutes. Once it comes to a boil, bring down the heat
a slow boil. The sauce should start bubbling and thickening. Cook for another 5 minutes, stirring almost constantly, until it has a thick, smooth,
melted cheese consistency.

Mix in the mustard and taste for salt. Serve hot or warm.

Spinach Linguine with Edamame Pesto

SERVES 4 • ACTIVE TIME: 15 MINUTES • TOTAL TIME: 30 MINUTES

(CAN BE MADE GLUTEN FREE IF USING GF PASTA)

No one should suffer a life without pesto, but a pesto without pine nuts or walnuts seems lifeless. So what's a girl to do? Once again, it's soybeans to the rescue! Edamame has just enough fat and texture to make a lighter, healthier pesto work. It also makes the pesto at once bulky and creamy. It's a miracle, really. Oh, little soybean, what can't you do? Here's pesto with linguine, sautéed mushrooms for meatiness, and red onions for just a tinge of sweetness. I'm sure this pesto will be making appearances elsewhere, too. It's not completely fat free, but it has about one-fifth the fat and calories of your average pesto plus five times the fiber. Not too shabby.

1 recipe **Edamame Pesto** (recipe follows)
8 ounces spinach linguine or other pasta
1 teaspoon olive oil
  Small red onion, cut into thinly sliced half-moons
½ pound cremini mushrooms, sliced
2 cloves garlic, minced
1 teaspoon dried thyme
¼ teaspoon salt
  Extra chopped fresh basil, for garnish

Put on a pot of salted water to boil. Then prepare the pesto.

Once the pesto is ready, preheat a large pan over medium heat. At this point your pasta water should be ready, so add the linguine.

Sauté the onion in oil for about 5 minutes. Use a little nonstick cooking spray as needed, or a splash of water if you prefer. Mix in the mushrooms, garlic, thyme, and salt. Cover the pot and cook for 5 more minutes, stirring occasionally.

The pasta should be ready now, so drain it.

When the mushrooms have cooked down, add the pasta to the pan, along with the pesto. Use a pasta spoon to stir and coat the linguine. Get everything good and mixed and the pesto heated through, about 3 minutes. The pesto should be relatively thick, but if it's too thick (not spreading out and coating the pasta) add a few tablespoons of water. Taste for salt.

Serve immediately, garnished with a little chopped fresh basil.

> ∾ **TIP** *As a cilantro lover, I like to sneak a handful into my pesto. It doesn't overwhelm, it just gives basil pesto a special little something. Try it if you like!* ∾

Edamame Pesto

SERVES 4 • ACTIVE TIME: 10 MINUTES • TOTAL TIME: 10 MINUTES

This makes a lot of pesto, meaning your pasta won't feel skimpy in the least, and your veggies will feel nice and smothered.

- 2 cloves garlic, chopped
- 1 cup packed basil leaves
- 1 (14-ounce) package frozen shelled edamame, thawed
- ½ cup vegetable broth
- 2 tablespoons freshly squeezed lemon juice
- 1 teaspoon olive oil
- ½ teaspoon salt
- 2 tablespoons nutritional yeast (optional)

**PER SERVING
(¼ RECIPE):**
Calories: 130
Calories from fat: 50
Total fat: 6 g
Saturated fat: 0 g
Trans fat: 0 g
Fiber: 5 g
Protein: 11 g
Cholesterol: 0 mg
Sodium: 370 mg
Vitamin A: 10%
Vitamin C: 25%
Calcium: 8%
Iron: 15%

Place the garlic and basil in a food processor and pulse a few times to get them chopped up. Add the remaining ingredients and blend until relatively smooth, scraping down the sides with a spatula to make sure you get everything. Add a little more vegetable broth if it seems too stiff. Set aside until ready to use.

Ginger Bok Choy & Soba

SERVES 2 TO 4 • ACTIVE TIME: 25 MINUTES • TOTAL TIME: 25 MINUTES

~~~~~~~~~~~~~~~~~~
PER SERVING
(¼ RECIPE):
Calories: 250
Calories from fat: 20
Total fat: 2 g
Saturated fat: 0 g
Trans fat: 0 g
Total carb: 51 g
Fiber: 5 g
Sugars: 4 g
Protein: 12 g
Cholesterol: 0 mg
Sodium: 930 mg
Vitamin A: 190%
Vitamin C: 160%
Calcium: 25%
Iron: 20%

I love bok choy because it's like two veggies in one: the crisp, bright stems and the silky, tender leaves. This dish is so simple yet so satisfying, especially on a weeknight when you want something green but steamed veggies are just not going to cut it. It's also great if you wanna slurp some noodles. The other thing I should mention is that it is extremely customizable. I sometimes add dry-fried tofu, prepared the same way as in the **Hoisin–Mustard Tofu** (page 153), or azuki beans or even black beans if I need something just a bit more hardy.

To have this on the table in under half an hour, boil the water for the soba first thing, and begin prepping the veggies. Start sautéing the veggies when you've added the soba to the water, for perfect timing. Per the directions, keep the bok choy leaves separate from the stems or all hell will break loose, because they're added at different times. Serve with extra soy sauce and Sriracha hot sauce.

   8 ounces soba noodles
   1 teaspoon peanut or vegetable oil
   1 bunch bok choy, leaves and stems separated, sliced across
     in ½-inch pieces (see tip page 187)
   1 small red onion, cut into thinly sliced half-moons
   4 cloves garlic, minced
   1 tablespoon minced fresh ginger
   ¼ teaspoon red pepper flakes
   1 tablespoon plus 1 teaspoon soy sauce

Prepare the soba noodles according to the package directions.

Preheat a large skillet over medium heat. Sauté the bok choy stems (not the leaves yet) and the onion in the oil for about 5 minutes, until the onion is translucent. Add the garlic, ginger, and red pepper flakes. Sauté for another minute or so. Add the bok choy leaves and soy sauce (and tofu or beans, if using.) Sauté for another minute, until the leaves are wilted.

By this time, the noodles should be ready. Add the drained noodles to the pan and sauté for about 2 minutes, using a pasta spoon, making sure everything is nice and coated. Serve immediately.

Pasta de los Angeles

SERVES 4 • ACTIVE TIME: 25 MINUTES • TOTAL TIME: 30 MINUTES

(CAN BE MADE GLUTEN FREE IF USING GF PASTA)

PER SERVING
(¼ RECIPE):
Calories: 440
Calories from fat: 30
Total fat: 3.5 g
Saturated fat: 0.5 g
Trans fat: 0 g
Fiber: 19 g
Protein: 24 g
Cholesterol: 0 mg
Sodium: 400 mg
Vitamin A: 250%
Vitamin C: 100%
Calcium: 20%
Iron: 45%

Pasta goes Mexican! That is, if you consider the flavors of black beans, cilantro, tomato, and lime to be Mexican. As for the recipe name, not only is this what angels are surely eating in heaven, but all these yummy flavors are tossed with quick-cooking angel hair pasta and a big bunch of spinach. So it's perfect for busy busy busy halo wearers who need a healthy dinner on the table like *now*.

8 ounces whole wheat angel hair pasta
1 teaspoon olive oil
1 cup thinly sliced shallot
3 cloves garlic
1 jalapeño, thinly sliced
1 cup chopped fresh cilantro, plus extra for garnish
4 plum tomatoes, chopped (about 3 cups)
½ teaspoon salt
   Zest and juice from 1 lime
1 (16-ounce) can black beans, drained and rinsed (about 1½ cups)
1 bunch spinach, coarse stems removed (about a pound), washed well

First, bring a covered pot of salted water to boil for the pasta. Then prepare the sauce.

Preheat a large skillet over medium heat. Sauté the shallot, garlic, and jalapeño in the oil for about 5 minutes. Stir in the cilantro and let cook for about a minute. Add the tomatoes, salt, and lime zest (reserve the juice). Cover the pan and cook for 10 more minutes, stirring occasionally. The tomatoes should be nicely broken down and saucy, but some whole pieces remaining are just fine. Add the black beans.

By this time the water should be ready. Add the pasta and cook according to the package directions.

While the pasta is cooking, add the spinach to the skillet, tossing to wilt. Once everything is added, cover and cook until the spinach is cooked down, about 3 more minutes. Squeeze in the lime juice. Turn off the heat.

When the pasta is ready, drain and add it to the pan. Use a pasta spoon to toss it, making sure that the pasta is well coated. Serve immediately, garnished with extra cilantro if you like.

∽ NUTRITION TIP One serving of this dish has 30 percent more protein than a 3-ounce serving of prime rib! We only need 10 to 15 percent of our total calories to come from protein, and black beans supply more than 20 percent. Even whole wheat pasta, long relegated to the carbohydrate category, is 12 percent protein. ∽

Lasagna with Roasted Cauliflower Ricotta & Spinach

SERVES 6 • ACTIVE TIME: 45 MINUTES • TOTAL TIME: 1½ HOURS

(CAN BE MADE GLUTEN FREE IF USING GF LASAGNA NOODLES)

Toasty, scrumptious roasted cauliflower blends perfectly into tofu ricotta and gives this lasagna so much flavor your head might burst. The sauce cooks right with the lasagna; no need for two billion pots and pans, only one million! A handful of olives is scattered across the top for that salty kick you need, so no expensive and fatty soy cheese required. I know the long cooking time can be scary sounding, but that's lasagna for you! To make things even easier, prep the ricotta a day ahead. It's actually an easy recipe to pull off and there is plenty of downtime. Be aware that this is baked in an 8-inch pan and it really fills it up to the top.

The possibilities for variations are endless but I'll list a few here:

- Instead of (or in addition to) olives, place thinly sliced fresh tomatoes on top.
- Tuck big cloves of roasted garlic into the layers (they sell them already roasted at many supermarkets); use about ¼ cup.
- Sauté some mushrooms and add them right under the spinach.
- Chop a roasted red pepper into the sauce.

ROASTED CAULIFLOWER RICOTTA:

- 1 medium-size head cauliflower (1½ to 2 pounds), chopped into ½-inch pieces
- 2 teaspoons olive oil
- ½ teaspoon salt
- 1 pound extra-firm tofu
- ¼ cup nutritional yeast flakes
- 2 tablespoons freshly squeezed lemon juice
  Several pinches of freshly ground black pepper

PER SERVING
(⅙ RECIPE):
Calories: 300
Calories from fat: 60
Total fat: 6 g
Saturated fat: 1 g
Trans fat: 0 g
Total carb: 49 g
Fiber: 8 g
Sugars: 9 g
Protein: 16 g
Cholesterol: 0 mg
Sodium: 670 mg
Vitamin A: 35%
Vitamin C: 150%
Calcium: 25%
Iron: 30%

RED SAUCE:

1 (28-ounce) can crushed tomatoes with basil
2 tablespoons chopped fresh thyme
3 cloves garlic, minced
½ teaspoon salt

TO ASSEMBLE:

8 ounces lasagna noodles, broken in half, cooked in salted water
1½ cups chopped fresh spinach
¼ cup chopped black olives

> **NOTE** It's kinda tough to find whole wheat lasagna noodles. The calculations here are for regular old lasagna noodles, but if you've got the gumption, Food Fight Grocery (www.foodfightgrocery.com) stocks whole wheat, and I bet if you begged your neighborhood health food store, they might carry them.

First, we'll roast the cauliflower. Preheat the oven to 400°F. Line a large, rimmed baking sheet with parchment paper; that way the cauliflower won't stick. Place the cauliflower on the sheet and drizzle the oil over it. Spray it with nonstick cooking spray and sprinkle with ¼ teaspoon of salt. Toss it with your hands to make sure everything is salted. Spread the cauliflower in a single layer and bake for 10 minutes, then flip it with a spatula. You don't have to flip each and every one, so don't get OCD about it. Bake for another 15 to 20 minutes, until lightly browned, tender, and toasty.

In the meantime, crumble the tofu into a mixing bowl. Use your hands to mash the tofu, squeezing it between your fingers, until it has the consistency of ricotta cheese. Add the nutritional yeast, lemon juice, pepper, and remaining salt. Use a fork to mix well.

> **NOTE** I think it's pretty common to find the crushed tomatoes with basil, but if you would prefer you can just add ¼ cup finely chopped basil to the sauce.

When the cauliflower is done, transfer it to the mixing bowl with the tofu mixture. Use a potato masher to mash it really well, for a minute or so. If it doesn't seem to be mashing enough with the potato masher, a few pulses in the food processor should get it nice and crumbly. Set aside.

To prepare the sauce, mix all its ingredients together and set aside.

Preheat the oven to 350°F. Pour a thin layer of red sauce on the bottom of an 8-inch square casserole. Line with a layer of noodles. Spread with one-third of the cauliflower ricotta. Layer with ¾ cup of spinach leaves. Pour on about a cup of sauce.

Repeat the process one more time, creating another identical layer, starting with the noodles. For the top layer it's just a little different: Layer with noodles, pour the sauce on first, then layer with ricotta. This layer doesn't get any spinach. Sprinkle with a layer of olives and press it into the the tofu.

Bake for 40 minutes, until the top is browned. You can serve it immediately or let it cool down for a bit first, whatever floats your boat!

> **NOTE** For time management, boil the water for the noodles about 10 minutes into the cauliflower roasting. Don't shut the oven off after roasting, just lower it to 350°F because you'll be cooking the lasagna noodles quickly after.

Miso Udon Stir-fry with Greens & Beans

SERVES 4 • ACTIVE TIME: 30 MINUTES • TOTAL TIME: 30 MINUTES

(CAN BE MADE GLUTEN FREE IF USING GF NOODLES)

~~~~~~~~~~~~~~~~~~~
PER SERVING
(¼ RECIPE):
Calories: 410
Calories from fat: 40
Total fat: 4.5 g
Saturated fat: 0 g
Trans fat: 0 g
Total carb: 75 g
Fiber: 12 g
Sugars: 9 g
Protein: 21 g
Cholesterol: 0 mg
Sodium: 1,310 mg
Vitamin A: 90%
Vitamin C: 210%
Calcium: 15%
Iron: 30%

Everything you want out of life in one bowl. Or at least everything you want out of dinner: filling udon noodles, beans, and greens with flavorful, salty miso. I love azuki beans here; they have a sweet and nutty flavor that cuddles right up to the miso. They also have a tendency to fall apart just a bit, which is great for coating the noodles. However, if you can't find azukis, black beans taste really great, too. For this recipe, use whatever miso you have on hand, but note that you may have to add more to your liking because misos vary in saltiness.

- 1 pound broccoli, stems sliced thinly, tops cut into florets
- 8 ounces brown rice udon noodles
- 1 teaspoon olive oil
- 6 cloves garlic, minced
- 1 bunch Swiss chard (about ½ pound), coarse stems removed, chopped roughly
- 1 cup thinly sliced green onions, plus extra for garnish
- ½ teaspoon salt
- 1 (16-ounce) can azuki beans, drained and rinsed
- ⅓ cup miso
- ½ cup hot water
- 4 teaspoons toasted sesame seeds
  Sriracha hot sauce, to serve

Prepare a pot of salted water for cooking the noodles.

Preheat a large skillet over medium-high heat. First, sauté the broccoli with a bit of nonstick cooking spray and a pinch of salt for about 5 minutes. Cover the pan and flip once or twice. The broccoli should be browned in some spots. Add a splash of water at the end, then cover for another minute. The pan should be steaming. Remove the broccoli from the pan and set aside. (By the way, that is my favorite way to prepare broccoli in general if I am serving it on the side.)

At this point, the water should be boiling. Use a mug to remove ½ cup of water; you can use that to mix into your miso in a few steps. Then cook the noodles according to the package directions. Drain when ready.

Now we'll put everything together. Preheat the large pan again, over medium heat. Sauté the garlic in the oil for about a minute, until fragrant. Add the chard, green onion, and salt, and sauté for about 5 minutes, until wilted. Add the beans and let heat through.

In the meantime, in a mug or measuring cup, mix together the miso and warm pasta water until relatively smooth.

Add the drained noodles to the pan, along with the miso mixture and broccoli. Sauté for about 2 minutes, using a pasta spoon, making sure everything is nice and coated. Taste for salt. To serve, top with sesame seeds and green onions and keep the Sriracha close at hand.

> ∾ NOTE You can use fresh udon noodles, which are often found in the refrigerated section of your supermarket, or you can use dried udon. Whatever is most convenient for you will work here; just follow the package directions to cook. ∾

Mac & Trees

SERVES 4 • ACTIVE TIME: 10 MINUTES • TOTAL TIME: 20 MINUTES

PER SERVING
(¼ RECIPE):
Calories: 330
Calories from fat: 30
Total fat: 3.5 g
Saturated fat: 0 g
Trans fat: 0 g
Total carb: 64 g
Fiber: 8 g
Sugars: 3 g
Protein: 13 g
Cholesterol: 0 mg
Sodium: 250 mg
Vitamin A: 15%
Vitamin C: 170%
Calcium: 6%
Iron: 15%

Nothing fancy here, but perfect weeknight fare when you want strong, comforting flavors, and some green, without too much effort. It doesn't get much easier than this! Start the sauce right after you start the water boiling, and you'll have this on the table in no time. In honor of my BFF Amy and our late night excursions to Brooklyn's vegan fast-food joint Food Swings, I like to drizzle plenty of cayenne hot sauce over it (Frank's Red Hot is my fave), or serve it with some **Buffalo Tempeh** (page 161) on top. If you'd like to bulk it up in a different direction, try a few slices of **Masala Baked Tofu** (page 146) tossed on top.

8 ounces brown rice macaroni
1 pound broccoli, tops cut into florets, stems chopped into
    ½-inch pieces
1 recipe **Easy Breezy Cheezy Sauce** (page 173)

Bring a pot of water to boil for the pasta and make your sauce.

Cook the pasta according to the package directions. About 5 minutes before you think the pasta will be done, add the broccoli to the pasta pot. When the pasta is ready, drain, and add back to the pot. Pour in the sauce and mix everything up. Serve!

Pasta e Fagioli with Spinach

SERVES 4 • ACTIVE TIME: 20 MINUTES • TOTAL TIME: 30 MINUTES

(CAN BE MADE GLUTEN-FREE IF USING GF PASTA)

Every recipe for pasta e fagioli will tell you that this is an Italian peasant dish, but I remember the first time I had pasta with beans I thought it was really fancy! This is a perfect, no-nonsense recipe for when you want your pasta, protein, and veggies all in one big bowl, and don't want to futz around too much.

- 1 teaspoon olive oil
- 6 cloves garlic, minced
- 2 pounds plum tomatoes, chopped roughly
- ¼ cup dry white wine or vegetable broth
- 1 teaspoon dried oregano
- 1 teaspoon dried thyme
- A few pinches of freshly ground black pepper
- 1 teaspoon salt
- 1 (15-ounce) can navy beans (about 1½ cups), drained and rinsed
- 8 ounces whole wheat small shells or orecchiette
- 1 pound baby spinach leaves, washed well

Bring a pot of water to boil for the pasta and preheat a large skillet over medium heat.

In the pan, sauté the garlic in oil for about 1 minute, until the garlic is fragrant. Add the tomatoes, wine, oregano, and salt. Bring to a boil. Once boiling, add the beans and then lower the heat to medium. Cook until the tomatoes are broken down and the sauce is reduced and thickened, about 15 minutes.

In the meantime, add the pasta to boiling water and cook according to the package directions. Once the sauce is thickened, simmer over low heat to keep warm.

Drain the pasta. In a bowl, alternate adding batches of pasta, beans, and spinach to the sauce, stirring with a pasta spoon to incorporate, until the spinach is completely wilted. Mix well and serve.

PER SERVING
(¼ RECIPE):
Calories: 440
Calories from fat: 30
Total fat: 3.5 g
Saturated fat: 0.5 g
Trans fat: 0 g
Total carb: 85 g
Fiber: 21 g
Sugars: 9 g
Protein: 23 g
Cholesterol: 0 mg
Sodium: 690 mg
Vitamin A: 250%
Vitamin C: 110%
Calcium: 25%
Iron: 45%

Curry Laksa

SERVES 4 • ACTIVE TIME: 30 MINUTES • TOTAL TIME: 30 MINUTES

(CAN BE MADE GLUTEN FREE IF USING GF TAMARI IN PLACE OF SOY SAUCE)

~~~~~~~~~~~~~~

PER SERVING
(¼ RECIPE):
Calories: 270
Calories from fat: 50
Total fat: 6 g
Saturated fat: 2 g
Trans fat: 0 g
Total carb: 50 g
Fiber: 3 g
Sugars: 12 g
Protein: 8 g
Cholesterol: 0 mg
Sodium: 570 mg
Vitamin A: 60%
Vitamin C: 100%
Calcium: 20%
Iron: 20%

I would probably get chased out of Malaysia if I got off the plane with a bowl of this and said it was Curry Laksa, but what it lacks in authenticity it makes up for in speed, ease, and healthfulness. Oh, and it tastes pretty darn good, too. If you like a big gigantic bowl of noodles, then this is your golden ticket. Noodles and tofu, mellow bok choy, and red peppers in a spicy, sweet, and sour red coconut milk broth. Serve with chopsticks and a big spoon.

This dish also makes really great leftovers! When left in the fridge, the tofu sucks up the curry and the lime flavor gets a little stronger. It even tastes great cold!

2 to 3	tablespoons red curry paste
1	small red onion, thinly sliced into half-moons
1	red pepper, seeded and sliced thinly (see tip)
1	tablespoon minced fresh ginger
2	cloves garlic, minced
1	bunch bok choy (prepared per tip)
4	cups vegetable broth
2	tablespoons soy sauce
½	teaspoon salt
1	block extra-firm tofu (about 14 ounces), cubed
8	ounces Pad Thai rice noodles
¾	cup light coconut milk
3	tablespoons lime juice (from 1 or 2 limes)
3	tablespoons agave
1	cup fresh cilantro, for garnish
	Extra lime wedges, for serving

Put a big pot of water on to boil for the noodles. In the meantime, prep all your veggies.

Preheat another 4-quart pot over medium high heat. Place 2 tablespoons of curry paste in the pot and mix in the onion and peppers. Sauté for about 2 minutes. Use a little nonstick cooking spray if it seems to be sticking excessively. Add the garlic and ginger, and sauté for another 2 minutes. Add the bok choy stems, water, soy sauce, and salt, and bring to a slow rolling boil (no need to cover). Add the tofu and cook for 10 more minutes.

At this point, your water for the noodles is probably boiling, so cook the noodles. They should be done in 5 minutes; drain and set aside.

Add the coconut milk, lime juice, and agave to the curry and mix, being gentle so as not to break the tofu. Taste for salt and spice. You may want to add up to another tablespoon of curry paste, depending on the strength of the brand you used.

To assemble, divide the bok choy leaves and place them in individual bowls. Use a pasta spoon to scoop the noodles. Ladle lots of curry in and garnish with a big old pile of cilantro and extra lime wedges.

∾ TIP To get really pretty red pepper slices, slice the pepper stem to bottom. Pull off the stem and pull out the seeds. Now slice the pepper widthwise, following its curve. You'll get pretty rainbow-shaped strips instead of boring old straight strips. ∾

∾ NOTE If using full-size bok choy, this is how I prepare it. I'm not crazy about leaving the stems very raw and snappy. I really like the flavor and texture better when it's well cooked. First, lob off about an inch of the bottom and toss it. Then separate all the leaves and wash them. Next, chop the stems up into ½-inch pieces and set them aside. You'll be left with leaves and the tender upper stem. Chop those into 2-inch pieces and keep them separate, because the stems are going to be added to the pot, but the leaves are going to be added to the bowl raw, where they'll wilt from the soup and become the perfect silky (but not mushy) texture. ∾

Creamy Mushroom Fettuccine

SERVES 4 • ACTIVE TIME: 15 MINUTES • TOTAL TIME: 30 MINUTES

(CAN BE MADE GLUTEN FREE IF USING GF FETTUCCINE)

Mushroom lovers rejoice! This pasta is nothing but slurp-worthy, creamy, earthy, mushroomy goodness. There's a little cheat in here to get things moving along with minimal effort, and that is a box of creamy portobello soup. But, you know, think of it more as a vegetable broth kind of help along. There are a few brands that make a vegan soup like this; I used Imagine brand.

8	ounces whole wheat fettuccine
1	teaspoon olive oil
5	cloves garlic, minced
½	pound cremini mushrooms, sliced ¼ inch thick
½	teaspoon salt
	Freshly ground black pepper
1½	teaspoons dried thyme
½	cup dry white wine
2	cups creamy portobello soup
2	tablespoons cornstarch
2	teaspoons balsamic vinegar
½	cup thinly sliced green onions

Bring a covered pot of salted water to boil for the pasta. Once boiling, add the pasta and cook according to the package directions.

Preheat a large skillet over medium heat. Sauté the garlic in the olive oil for about a minute, being careful not to burn it. Add the mushrooms to the pan, along with the salt, pepper, and thyme. Sauté for about 5 minutes until a lot of moisture has released.

Add the white wine and turn up the heat to bring it to a boil. Let the liquid reduce by about half, which will take 5 minutes or so.

In the meantime, pour the soup into a measuring cup and stir in the cornstarch vigorously, until pretty well dissolved. Add this mixture to the pan, lower the heat to medium, and let it thicken for about 5 more minutes. Your pasta should be cooking by now, too.

Once thickened, turn off the heat and add the balsamic vinegar. When the pasta is ready, drain it and add it to the pan. Stir well and let it sit for a few minutes to absorb the flavors. Taste for salt and seasonings.

To serve, transfer the mushroom fettuccine to bowls and top with sliced green onions.

Cajun Beanballs & Spaghetti

SERVES 4 • ACTIVE TIME: 30 MINUTES • TOTAL TIME: 1 HOUR

(CAN BE MADE GLUTEN FREE IF USING GF TAMARI IN PLACE OF SOY SAUCE; GF CRACKERS IN PLACE OF BREAD CRUMBS; AND GF SPAGHETTI)

PER SERVING
(¼ RECIPE):
Calories: 450
Calories from fat: 45
Total fat: 5 g
Saturated fat: 1 g
Trans fat: 0 g
Total carb: 87 g
Fiber: 17 g
Sugars: 11 g
Protein: 23 g
Cholesterol: 0 mg
Sodium: 790 mg
Vitamin A: 70%
Vitamin C: 60%
Calcium: 25%
Iron: 35%

They say that black-eyed peas bring you luck when eaten on New Year's Day, and New Year's is also the time of year many people go vegan, so not only will you be lucky, so will the animals! I love a couple of big meatballs over supersaucy and slurpy spaghetti. This version pays homage to Louisiana with some Cajun spices, hot sauce, and a smattering of scallions. Make sure to bulk up your pasta with some veggies (see page 164 for ideas). In this recipe we use zucchini, but you can use any veggies you like, or use one of the veggieful marinara options (page 194).

1 recipe **Spicy Cajun Marinara** (page 195)
12 Black-Eyed Pea and Tempeh Beanballs (recipe follows)
8 ounces whole wheat spaghetti
2 cups zucchini, cut into thin half-moons
1 cup thinly sliced scallions

I realize there are a lot of recipes within a recipe here, so let me just tell you how to get this done quickly and efficiently. Prepare the marinara first. Once you've got that going, start the meatballs. When the meatballs are in the oven, start the water for the pasta.

Cook the pasta according to the package directions. In the last 3 minutes of cooking, add the zucchini to the pot.

Drain the pasta and zucchini, then add them back to the pot. Pour in the marinara sauce and mix well. Toss in the beanballs to coat. Transfer to individual bowls and top with three beanballs each. Scatter the scallions over the top. Serve!

> ∾ NOTE *This is a lot of food, so expect leftovers! To make this gluten free, use crushed GF crackers instead of the bread crumbs in the beanballs and use a gluten-free tamari for the soy sauce. And, of course, gluten-free spaghetti.* ∾

Black-Eyed Pea & Tempeh Beanballs

MAKES 20 BEANBALLS, 3 PER SERVING • ACTIVE TIME: 20 MINUTES •
TOTAL TIME: 45 MINUTES

**(CAN BE MADE GLUTEN FREE IF USING GF TAMARI IN PLACE OF SOY SAUCE
AND GF CRACKERS IN PLACE OF BREAD CRUMBS)**

This recipe makes twenty beanballs, so that once you've eaten them on your spaghetti, you'll have a few left over to do what you please with. Try them in a wrap or on top of a salad.

12	ounces tempeh
1	(15-ounce) can black-eyed peas
2	cloves garlic
1	teaspoon dried thyme
2	teaspoons dried oregano
½	teaspoon paprika
	Several pinches of freshly ground black pepper
1	tablespoon soy sauce
1	tablespoon tomato paste
1	tablespoon balsamic vinegar
¼	cup whole wheat bread crumbs
¼	teaspoon salt

PER SERVING
(3 BEANBALLS):
Calories: 170
Calories from fat: 20
Total fat: 2.5 g
Saturated fat: 0 g
Trans fat: 0 g
Total carb: 28 g
Fiber: 8 g
Sugars: 3 g
Protein: 10 g
Cholesterol: 0 mg
Sodium: 260 mg
Vitamin A: 35%
Vitamin C: 4%
Calcium: 15%
Iron: 8%

First, prepare a steamer to steam the tempeh. Once the steamer is ready, break the tempeh into bite-size pieces and steam for 10 minutes.

In the meantime, preheat the oven to 350°F and line a large cookie sheet with parchment paper.

In a mixing bowl, use a fork or mini potato masher or avocado masher to mash the beans. They should be well mashed, with no whole beans left, but not completely smooth like a puree. Use a Microplane grater to grate in the garlic (if you don't have one, just mince it really well). Add the herbs and spices, soy sauce, tomato paste, and balsamic vinegar, and mix well.

When the tempeh is ready, add it to the mixture and mash well. It's good if it's still steaming hot because that will help all the flavors meld before baking. When the mixture is cool enough to handle (a few minutes), add the bread crumbs and salt. Taste for salt (the batter may be a bit bitter; it will mellow out when baked).

Using about 2 tablespoons of the mixture per ball, roll the mixture into walnut-size balls, placing them on the baking pan. Spray with an ample amount of nonstick cooking spray and cover loosely with tinfoil. Bake for 15 minutes, flip the balls, and bake for 10 more minutes, uncovered.

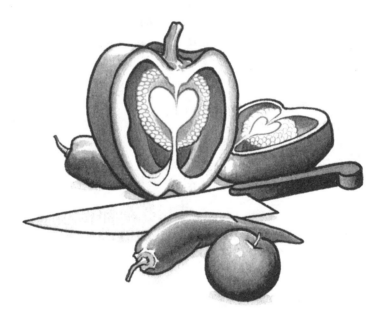

Mom's Marinara

MAKES 4 CUPS, SERVES 4 • ACTIVE TIME: 10 MINUTES • TOTAL TIME:
20 MINUTES

All people need a reliable, basic marinara sauce in their arsenal. There really is no reason in the world to buy jarred pasta sauce, with all that added sugar and who knows what else. This version uses a healthy dose of garlic and a touch of your usual marinara suspects, thyme and oregano, to give it that Brooklyn Italian mom taste. It's marinara sauce; I don't need to sell it. I bet it could make an old sneaker taste good (a vegan sneaker, please)! Once you get the basics down, try some of the variations. There never needs to be a dull pasta night!

1   teaspoon olive oil
3   cloves garlic, minced
1   teaspoon dried thyme
1   teaspoon dried oregano
    Freshly ground black pepper
1   (24-ounce) can crushed tomatoes
½   teaspoon salt

~~~~~~~~~~~~~~~~
PER SERVING
(1 CUP):
Calories: 70
Calories from fat: 15
Total fat: 1.5 g
Saturated fat: 0 g
Trans fat: 0 g
Total carb: 13 g
Fiber: 3 g
Sugars: 4 g
Protein: 3 g
Cholesterol: 0 mg
Sodium: 520 mg
Vitamin A: 25%
Vitamin C: 30%
Calcium: 6%
Iron: 15%

Preheat a 2-quart pot over medium-low heat. Sauté the garlic in the oil for about a minute. Add the thyme, oregano, and pepper, and sauté for a minute more, adding a splash of water if necessary. Add the tomatoes and salt, and stir everything together. Cover the pot, leaving a little gap for steam to escape, and cook for 10 minutes. Taste for salt and seasoning and serve!

VARIATIONS

Spicy Marinara:

Use this in conjunction with any variation—just add ½ teaspoon red pepper flakes along with garlic.

Marinara Olivada:

Add ¼ cup chopped kalamata olives when you add the garlic. Proceed with recipe.

ADDS 15 CALORIES, 1.5 GRAMS OF FAT, AND 150 MG OF SODIUM PER SERVING.

Marinara Puttanesca:

Along with the kalamata olives (above), add ½ cup capers.

ADDS 20 CALORIES, 1.5 GRAMS OF FAT, AND 525 MG SODIUM PER SERVING.

Cauli Marinara:

After preheating pan, add 3 cups chopped cauliflower and spray lightly with nonstick cooking spray. Cover the pan and cook for about 5 minutes, stirring often. Add a splash of veggie broth and cover, letting the pan steam for 30 seconds. Push the cauliflower to the side, sauté the garlic as directed, and proceed with the recipe.

ADDS 18 CALORIES, 2 GRAMS OF FIBER, ZERO FAT, AND 20 MG SODIUM PER SERVING.

Mushroom Marinara:

After preheating the marinara, sauté 16 ounces finely chopped cremini mushrooms in the oil. Add splashes of water if it seems dry. Stir in the garlic and proceed with the recipe.

ADDS 30 CALORIES, 1 GRAM OF FIBER, AND ZERO FAT AND SODIUM PER SERVING.

Roasted Red Pepper Marinara:

When you add the tomatoes, also add a finely chopped roasted red pepper (about ½ cup if you use jarred).

ADDS 8 CALORIES, 1 GRAM OF FIBER, AND ZERO FAT AND SODIUM PER SERVING.

Sautéed Onion Marinara:

Before adding the garlic, sauté a small, finely chopped onion for about 5 minutes. Add splashes of water if things appear dry. Proceed with recipe.

ADDS 10 CALORIES AND ZERO FAT AND SODIUM PER SERVING.

Spicy Cajun Marinara:

Add ½ teaspoon red pepper flakes along with the garlic, add 1 tablespoon Cajun spice blend along with the tomatoes, and add hot sauce at the end, to taste.

THE CAJUN BLEND DOES NOT ADD ANY CALORIES OR FAT, BUT MAY ADD SODIUM, DEPENDING ON THE BRAND.

Lentil Bolognese:

In a covered 2-quart pot, bring 1 cup red lentils, 2 cups water, and a pinch of salt to a boil. Once boiling, lower to a simmer and cook for about 20 minutes, until the lentils are tender and the water is mostly absorbed. Prepare the marinara recipe as directed, adding the cooked lentils when you add the tomatoes.

ADDS 165 CALORIES, 5.5 GRAMS OF FIBER, 1 GRAM OF FAT, AND 5 MG OF SODIUM PER SERVING.

Eggplant Marinara:

Cut 1¼ pounds eggplant into ½-inch chunks. Sauté the garlic as directed, and add the eggplant with ¼ cup vegetable broth and a pinch of salt. Sauté for about 5 minutes to get the eggplant a bit softer. Add the remaining ingredients and cook until the eggplant is thoroughly tender, about 20 minutes.

ADDS 35 CALORIES, 5 GRAMS OF FIBER, ZERO FAT, AND 30 MG OF SODIUM PER SERVING.

Marinara with Peas:

Yes, this is simple, but it's also so yummy. Just add 2 cups of frozen peas along with the tomatoes, and proceed with the recipe.

ADDS 60 CALORIES, ZERO FAT, AND 50 MG OF SODIUM PER SERVING.

CHAPTER 7

Soul-Satisfying Soups

YOU KNOW THAT IMAGE OF A CHEF LEANING OVER THE STOVE, fanning the steam from his simmering pot toward his face, eyes closed and blissful as he inhales his creation? There's probably soup in that pot.

You can learn a lot about cooking from making a pot of soup. You'll hone your knife skills by mincing garlic and dicing onion and veggies. And you'll get to know each and every vegetable—the soups in this chapter cover just about everything you're likely to find in the produce aisle. By the time you're through, rutabaga shouldn't be an alien-looking potato. Get familiar with herbs and you'll impress your friends and family by being able to tell the difference between flat-leaf parsley and cilantro without having to smell them. I guarantee that after a few batches of soup you'll be gliding through your kitchen, seasoning to your taste, adding a little of this, a little of that.

Much has been made over soup and weight loss. There have got to be about fifty books dedicated to the subject. But the idea is pretty simple: load up on vegetables, beans, grains, and water instead of on heavier foods. Soup is the perfect vehicle for this. If you're just easing into a plant-based diet, or you just aren't all that used to eating vegetables that aren't popcorn and onion rings, then this chapter would be a great place to start.

Lotsa Veggies Lentil Soup

SERVES 6 • ACTIVE TIME: 15 MINUTES • TOTAL TIME: 1 HOUR

Lentil soup been slung from the stove top of everyone from the ancient Egyptians to the present-day blogger, and with good reason. Its quick cooking time, nourishing flavor, and hearty texture are just the beginning: lentils also have the highest protein content of any plant-based food. And just as the Egyptians gave us the building blocks for society, this soup gives you the building blocks for a super-healthy and filling soup, using pantry items and a few staple veggies.

Sauté your onion and garlic while chopping the rest of the veggies and the prep time is hardly anything. Then once the pot gets going, tide yourself over with a few stolen carrots, catch up on your e-mails, or leave scathing comments on conservative blogs all while basking in the steamy aroma of a simmering pot of soup. Throwing a few handfuls of spinach in at the end is a great trick to up the fiber and nutrition content of any soup. It's so good you'll want to be buried in your pyramid with it, or at least keep a container of it in the freezer at all times.

- 1 teaspoon olive oil
- 1 medium-size onion, cut into medium dice
- 3 cloves garlic, minced
- 2 teaspoons dried thyme
- 1 teaspoon dried tarragon
  Several pinches of freshly ground black pepper
- ½ teaspoon sea salt
- 2 ribs celery, diced small
- ½ pound carrots, diced small
- ½ pound zucchini, diced small
- 1 cup French lentils (green lentils are fine, too)
- 6 cups vegetable broth
- 6 ounces tomato sauce
- ¼ pound spinach leaves, washed well and chopped (about 3 cups)

Preheat a 4-quart pot over medium heat. Sauté the onion in the oil for about 5 minutes, until translucent. Use a little nonstick cooking spray if needed. Add the garlic, thyme, tarragon, pepper, and salt, and sauté for another minute.

Add the celery, carrots, zucchini, lentils, and vegetable broth, and mix to combine. Cover the pot and bring to a boil. Once boiling, lower the heat to a simmer and cook for about 45 minutes, until the lentils and veggies are very tender and the soup is thickened.

Add the tomato sauce and spinach, and cook until the spinach is wilted. You can serve it immediately, but as with most soups it's better if you let it sit for at least 10 minutes first, and it tastes even better the next day.

INGREDIENT SCAVENGER HUNT

I use a plethora of lentils throughout the book, but this recipe calls for french lentils, also called du Puy lentils or, if you really want to be a snob about it, or you are French, lentilles du Puy. Hailing from central France, they're a smaller and firmer lentil that I prefer to use when I'm craving something really hearty and, dare I say, meaty. You probably won't find them in the average grocery store, but Whole Foods Market–type stores are sure to have them in stock. You can also find them in the sort of store that might say "gourmet" on the awning, but "gourmet" doesn't have to mean expensive. If the price is exorbitant, grab regular old green lentils and don't look back; the soup will still be fabulous.

Ceci-Roasted Red Pepper Soup

SERVES 4 • ACTIVE TIME: 10 MINUTES • TOTAL TIME: 45 MINUTES

PER SERVING
(¼ RECIPE):
Calories: 170
Calories from fat: 30
Total fat: 3.5 g
Saturated fat: 0 g
Trans fat: 0 g
Total carb: 28 g
Fiber: 7 g
Sugars: 10 g
Protein: 8 g
Cholesterol: 0 mg
Sodium: 830 mg
Vitamin A: 50%
Vitamin C: 150%
Calcium: 8%
Iron: 15%

I've got no quarrel with consuming red bell peppers as is. They're all fair and well when you need something to dip in your hummus. But roasting red peppers makes them sweet and exotic-tasting, taking them well out of the crudité realm and into serious cuisine. So serious in fact that I had to give the soup a vaguely Italian name. Ceci means "chickpea," and here they are partially blended with the roasted peppers and fresh tomatoes to give the soup a great texture that'll keep you saying "mmm" in Italian, spoonful after spoonful.

2 large red bell peppers
1 medium-size onion, chopped finely
3 cloves garlic, minced
2 teaspoons dried rosemary
½ teaspoon salt
  Freshly ground black pepper
1 pound tomatoes, chopped roughly (3 average-size; about 2 cups)
1 teaspoon ground coriander
3 cups vegetable broth
1 (15-ounce) can chickpeas, drained and rinsed

To roast the peppers, preheat the oven to 375°F, cut out the stem with a paring knife, and discard it along with the seeds. Stand the peppers in a small baking pan (a pie plate or bread pan works great). Bake for about 35 minutes. They should be really soft; they might even collapse a bit. Remove from the oven, and store (see tip) or use a fork and knife to chop them into bite-size pieces (because they'll be too hot to touch). If storing overnight, chop into bite-size pieces when ready to make soup.

In a skillet, sauté the onion in the oil for about 5 minutes, until translucent. Use a little nonstick cooking spray if needed. Add the garlic, rosemary, salt and black pepper, and sauté for another minute. Mix in the tomatoes, stirring constantly for about a minute. The tomato should deglaze the pan.

Add the coriander, vegetable broth, and chickpeas; stir and cover. Bring to a low boil and cook covered for about 15 minutes, stirring occasionally. You just want the tomatoes to break down and the flavors to meld.

Add the roasted peppers. Use an immersion blender to blend about half of the soup or transfer half of the soup to a blender and puree, then add it back to the pot. If you're using a blender, be careful not to let steam build up while you blend; just do a few pulses, then lift the lid to let steam escape.

> ∾ NUTRITION TIP *One red bell pepper has more than twice the vitamin C of an orange, more than three times your daily needs.* ∾

Let the soup sit for a few minutes, taste for salt, and serve.

> ∾ TIP *To have this dish come together in a flash, roast the peppers the night before. Place them in a sealed plastic bag and refrigerate. They'll be ready to use when you want them! Alternatively, you can roast the peppers, then get the soup started. Once the peppers are done, it will be just about time to add them to the soup.* ∾

Butternut-Apple Soup

SERVES 6 • ACTIVE TIME: 15 MINUTES • TOTAL TIME: 45 MINUTES

~~~~~~~~~~
PER SERVING
(⅙ RECIPE):
Calories: 200
Calories from fat: 10
Total fat: 1.5 g
Saturated fat: 0 g
Trans fat: 0 g
Total carb: 41 g
Fiber: 7 g
Sugars: 16 g
Protein: 3 g
Cholesterol: 0 mg
Sodium: 390 mg
Vitamin A: 490%
Vitamin C: 90%
Calcium: 15%
Iron: 15%

This is the soup that gets me through autumn and winter. From apple-picking season until daffodils start poking out of the garden (well, everyone else's garden), you will find a pot of this soup simmering on my stove every week. Flavored with rosemary, ginger, lime, and just a little bit of spice, it's the perfect cold-weather pick-me-up. If you don't have any apple cider, then apple juice works, or you can even use water and a little agave at the end if it needs it. If you like, experiment with different squashes such as acorn, dumpling, or good old pumpkin. If you use delicata, you don't need to peel the skin, so that's a plus. You can also use pears in place of apples for a change of pace.

1 teaspoon olive oil

1 medium-size onion, diced small

1 tablespoon minced fresh ginger

3 cloves garlic, minced

½ teaspoon red pepper flakes

2 teaspoons dried rosemary

½ teaspoon salt

3 pounds butternut squash, peeled, seeded, and cut into ¾-inch chunks

1 pound red apples, peeled, cored, and cut into ¾-inch slices

2 cups apple cider

2 cups vegetable broth

1 tablespoon freshly squeezed lime juice

> ⤻ TIP *To make quick work of the butternut squash, stand it up and peel it. Then, use a chef's knife to cut the round part off. Slice the round part in half, and use a tablespoon to scrape out the seeds and stringy bits. Proceed to cut into chunks. Get this down and you should be able to prep a butternut in under 5 minutes.* ⤻

Preheat a 4-quart pot over medium heat. Sauté the onions in the oil for 5 to 7 minutes, until translucent.

Add the ginger and garlic, red pepper flakes, rosemary, and salt, and sauté for a minute more. Add the squash, apples, apple cider, and broth. Cover and bring to a boil. Once boiling, lower the heat just a bit and simmer briskly for about 20 more minutes, or until the squash is tender.

Puree the soup using either an immersion blender or by transferring half the soup at a time to a food processor or blender in batches. If you prefer, you can leave the soup a little chunky by only pureeing half or so. If using a blender, be sure to let the steam escape so that it doesn't build up in the blender.

Add the lime juice and season to taste. Serve!

Bistro Broccoli Chowder

SERVES 6 • ACTIVE TIME: 15 MINUTES • TOTAL TIME: 45 MINUTES

Broccoli soup is thickened with potato and peppery parsnips, and made creamy with a bit of almond milk. It's the kind of soup that would go great with a baked tofu sandwich and a salad, and if vegan bistros existed, I bet they would serve something like this. I use unsweetened almond milk, but if you like, you can use soy. Just don't use anything sweetened or it will taste out of place. Make it my way once, but you can really mess around with this recipe, using other vegetables—cauliflower, asparagus, and zucchini are all contenders—and spicing to your liking. I'm just using simple rosemary here, but you can try thyme and dill as well. If you don't have a parsnip, just use extra potato or carrot. The phrase, "The world is yours!" comes to mind, only replace world with soup. Serve in teacups so it really feels like you're eating in a bistro!

1 medium-size onion, diced small

4 cloves garlic

1 teaspoon dried rosemary
  Several pinches of freshly ground black pepper

½ teaspoon salt

1 pound Yukon Gold potatoes, cut into ½-inch chunks (no need to peel)

½ pound parsnips, peeled and cut into slightly less than ½-inch chunks

5 cups chopped broccoli, the stalks chopped into thin slices, the tops cut into small florets

4 cups vegetable broth

1 cup unsweetened almond milk

Preheat a 4-quart pot over medium heat. Sauté the onion in the olive oil for 5 to 7 minutes, until softened. Add the garlic, rosemary, pepper, and salt, and cook for a minute more. Pour in the vegetable broth and add the potatoes and parsnips. Cover and bring to a boil. Once boiling, lower the heat and let simmer for 10 minutes. Add the broccoli and cook for 20 more minutes.

Add the almond milk and heat through. Use an immersion blender to blend about half the soup, keeping it a bit chunky. If you don't have an immersion blender (get one!), then transfer about half of the soup to a blender and puree, then add it back to the soup. If you're using a blender, be careful not to let the steam build up while you blend.

Taste for salt and seasoning, and serve.

> ∾ TIP *For a pretty garnish, and to add a little crunch to your soup, chop up a broccoli floret into very fine crumbs and sprinkle it over cups of soup.* ∾

Arabian Lentil & Rice Soup

SERVES 6 • ACTIVE TIME: 15 MINUTES • TOTAL TIME: ABOUT AN HOUR

G S D

PER SERVING
(⅙ RECIPE):
Calories: 230
Calories from fat: 20
Total fat: 2.5 g
Saturated fat: 0 g
Trans fat: 0 g
Total carb: 40 g
Fiber: 12 g
Sugars: 5 g
Protein: 12 g
Cholesterol: 0 mg
Sodium: 960 mg
Vitamin A: 100%
Vitamin C: 20%
Calcium: 6%
Iron: 20%

They don't call Portland "Little Lebanon," but maybe they should! There is a large Lebanese community and so many wonderful Lebanese restaurants here, all with a clearly marked vegan menu. This soup was inspired by one of those restaurants. Creamy red lentils with fragrant brown basmati make a complete meal, perfect for a weeknight where you don't feel like having lots of pots on the stove. A healthy dose of lemon brings out the the sultry flavors of cumin. Definitely taste for seasoning at the end to adjust to your liking.

Typically these Lebanese restaurants offer baked pita fresh from the oven straight to your table. It's the size of a giant Frisbee and the server flops it over a little cast-iron stand. But why don't you make do with a little whole wheat pita?

2 teaspoons olive oil

1 medium-size onion, diced small

6 cloves garlic, minced

Several pinches of freshly ground black pepper

1 teaspoon salt

1 tablespoon ground cumin

1 teaspoon ground coriander

1½ cups small-diced carrots

1 cup dried red lentils

½ cup brown basmati rice

1 teaspoon lemon zest

6 cups vegetable broth

¼ cup freshly squeezed lemon juice

Preheat a 4-quart pot over medium-high heat. Sauté the onions in the oil until translucent, about 4 minutes. Add the garlic, pepper, and salt and sauté for another minute. Add the spices and stir continuously for about 15 seconds to toast them a bit.

Add the carrots, lentils, rice, zest, and broth. Cover the pot and bring to a boil, keeping a close eye on it. Once it's boiling, lower the heat to a simmer and cook for about 40 minutes, until the lentils are creamy and the rice is tender. Depending on the rice you use, it could be 15 minutes, more or less. Stir occasionally to prevent the soup from burning at the bottom. If necessary, thin the soup with water. Add the lemon juice. Taste for salt and seasonings.

Let the soup sit for 10 minutes or so for maximum flavor, and serve.

❧ INGREDIENT SCAVENGER HUNT

More fun with lentils! Red lentils are actually beautifully coral hued when dry. As they cook they turn yellow and creamy. They don't remain whole like green lentils; instead expect a velvety smooth base for your soup, more like split pea, really. They shouldn't be hard to find; if your supermarket has any sort of dried bean section, it will most likely carry red lentils. If you absolutely must, split peas make an appropriate substitute in this soup. ❧

Tortilla Soup

SERVES 6 • ACTIVE TIME: 15 MINUTES • TOTAL TIME: 30 MINUTES

Tortilla soup is one of those things that I absolutely crave, and luckily this version comes together in half an hour, so I don't end up scratching anyone's eyes out, as I usually do when I crave something that I can't have. For me, the perfect tortilla soup has a lighter tomato broth (no tomato paste here) and simple but assertive spice. And here's a PSA: Tortilla soup isn't simply chili with some crushed chips on top of it! For a full-bodied soup, adding crushed tortilla chips while the soup is cooking is the way to go. A sprinkle of crushed chips on the top finishes it off for a perfect fiesta of flavor and texture.

Baked tortilla chips provide the best nutrition profile, but regular ones will work, too; it's not like there are a ton of them in here. A poblano gives more authentic flavor, but a plain old green pepper is just fine. This recipe is one that you shouldn't need to read again once you've made it once or twice, because you don't need to measure much; even the vegetable broth is measured out in the can of tomatoes that you use.

1   teaspoon olive oil
1   small onion, sliced thinly
2   jalapeños, seeded and sliced thinly
1   poblano pepper or green bell pepper, seeded and chopped
    into ½-inch pieces
4   cloves garlic, minced
¼   teaspoon red pepper flakes (optional, if you like it extra spicy)
1   teaspoon salt
24 ounces whole tomatoes
24 ounces vegetable broth
4   ounces baked tortilla chips (about 2 cups)
1   tablespoon ground cumin
1   (15-ounce) can pinto beans, drained and rinsed
1   cup frozen corn
½   cup chopped fresh cilantro, plus extra for garnish
    Juice from 1 lime

Preheat a 4-quart pot over medium-high heat. Sauté the onions, jalapeños, and poblano pepper in the oil until the onions are translucent, about 5 minutes. Use a little nonstick cooking spray or broth if needed. Add the garlic, red pepper flakes, and salt, and sauté for another minute.

Break up the tomatoes with your fingers and add them to the pot, including the juice. Fill the tomato can with the vegetable broth and add that to the pot. Mix in the cumin. Crush 2 ounces of the chips into crumbs (some bigger pieces are okay) and add to the pot. Cover and bring to a boil. Once boiling, lower the heat to a simmer, add the beans, corn, and cilantro, and let simmer for 5 more minutes.

Add the lime juice and taste for salt and seasoning. Ladle the soup into bowls, crumble the remaining tortilla chips over the top, garnish with cilantro, and serve.

∾ NUTRITION TIP

The combination of vitamin C and the type of iron found in plant-based foods, called nonheme iron, significantly increases iron absorption. Iron is a crucial nutrient, especially for vegetarians and vegans. Interestingly, studies show that vegans consume more iron and have better iron levels than do vegetarians. ∾

Cauliflower Pesto Soup

SERVES 4 • ACTIVE TIME: 10 MINUTES • TOTAL TIME: ABOUT 25 MINUTES

PER SERVING
(WITHOUT PINE NUTS)
(¼ RECIPE):
Calories: 50
Calories from fat: 10
Total fat: 1.5 g
Saturated fat: 0 g
Trans fat: 0 g
Total carb: 11 g
Fiber: 3 g
Sugars: 5 g
Protein: 5 g
Cholesterol: 0 mg
Sodium: 880 mg
Vitamin A: 10%
Vitamin C: 90%
Calcium: 8%
Iron: 8%
If you use the pine
nuts, you will have
20 more calories and
2 more grams of fat
per serving.

Inspired by a big old bowl of pesto, this soup gets you there without all the fatty nuts and oily oils. Basil and cauliflower are pureed, and garnished with a little more basil and some toasted pine nuts. Its simple flavors are more reminiscent of something you'd order in a trattoria in Venice than of a big sloppy cup of soup in downtown Manhattan, so light some candles, unfold your finest linen tablecloth, and sip away like the refined individual you are. Oh, and although it might be tempting to eat all those pine nuts in one big bite, resist the urge and try to savor them throughout the soup. If you'd prefer something with less fat, you can omit the nuts, though. Serve with some bread or a nice big entrée salad.

1 teaspoon olive oil
4 cloves garlic, minced
1 head cauliflower (about a pound), leaves removed,
   cut into florets
4 cups broth
½ teaspoon salt
   Freshly ground black pepper
1 tablespoon arrowroot powder
1 cup loosely packed fresh basil leaves, plus a little extra
   for garnish
6 teaspoons toasted pine nuts (optional)

Preheat a 4-quart pot over medium heat. Sauté the garlic in the olive oil for about a minute, being careful not to let it burn. Add the cauliflower, 3 cups of the broth (alert! only three! you'll be adding the last cup in a bit), salt, and several pinches of pepper. Cover the pot and bring it to a boil. Let cook, stirring every now and again, for about 10 minutes, or until the cauliflower is tender.

Vigorously mix together the final cup of broth and the arrowroot until dissolved. Lower heat a bit so that the soup is at a slow boil. Mix in the arrowroot mixture and cook uncovered for another 5 minutes until slightly thickened. Add the basil leaves and remove from heat. Use an immersion blender to puree until smooth. Taste for salt.

If you don't have a immersion blender (get one!), then use a blender or a food processor to puree it in batches, being careful to lift the lid once in a while so that the steam doesn't build up and explode.

Serve the soup garnished with chopped fresh basil and a teaspoon of pine nuts. To garnish, carefully place a little pile of basil on the soup, and then rest the pine nuts on the basil. If it sinks, oh well! It will taste just as yummy.

TIP *The cauliflower is getting pureed, so don't worry about chopping the florets in uniform-size pieces. Just have at it; it shouldn't take more than 2 minutes to chop. And when you puree, really puree! Don't be lazy about it. Get it really smooth and creamy.*

⁓ INGREDIENT SCAVENGER HUNT

Pine nuts (also called pignolis) can be super pricy, so buy them in the bulk section of your health food superstore and save a few bucks. Buying in bulk lets you control how much you purchase, so if you're only planning on using ¼ cup, that's all you need to buy. I store mine in the freezer to keep them fresh and then toast them as needed. It seems crazy that they're so expensive but if you think about how they're cultivated, you'll understand why. They really do grow in pine cones! Thus the name. But don't go raiding the woods in search of tonight's dinner; there are only a few species that grow pine nuts and they are generally farmed. Stick with the bulk bins.

• To toast pine nuts, preheat a small sauté pan over low heat. Add the pine nuts and stir often for about 4 minutes, or until the pine nuts are dark and toasty. Remove from heat immediately. A good time to toast 'em in this recipe is when the cauliflower is boiling. ⁓

Caldo Verde with Crumbled Tempeh

SERVES 6 • ACTIVE TIME: 20 MINUTES • TOTAL TIME: 45 MINUTES

Every country seems to have a version of potatoes and greens—caldo verde is Portugal's offering. Although it's traditionally flavored with sausage, we're using some braised tempeh tossed in at the end and fennel seed for that sausage-y flavor. I love this recipe because it's got everything you need to make a complete dinner, it's the "meat and potatoes" of soups, only with a healthy dose of green thrown in. If you're just easing into the world of leafy greens, then this is a delicious and easy way to do it. I used green chard (because, you know, verde means "green"), but you can use lacinato kale, regular kale, or even cabbage.

SOUP:

1 teaspoon olive oil
1 small onion, diced small
3 cloves garlic, minced
1½ teaspoons fennel seeds, crushed
1 teaspoon dried thyme
½ teaspoon red pepper flakes
Several pinches of freshly ground black pepper
½ teaspoon salt
4 cups vegetable broth
1½ pounds Yukon Gold potatoes, scrubbed and cut into ½-inch chunks
1 bunch chard, coarse stems removed, shredded (see tip)

TEMPEH:

1 (8-ounce) package tempeh
2 tablespoons tamari
½ teaspoon olive oil
1 tablespoon freshly squeezed lemon juice

PREPARE THE SOUP:

Preheat a 4-quart pot over medium heat. Sauté the onion in the olive oil for 5 to 7 minutes, until softened. Use nonstick cooking spray if needed. Add the garlic, fennel, thyme, red pepper flakes, a few pinches of black pepper, and the salt, and cook for a minute more. Pour in the vegetable broth and add the potatoes. Cover and bring to a boil. Once boiling, lower the heat and let simmer (still covered) for about 20 minutes, or until the potatoes are tender. In the meantime, make the tempeh (directions to follow).

> **TIP** To shred the chard, remove the coarse stems, then layer the chard leaves into a pile. Roll the pile up into a tube, then thinly slice.

Use an immersion blender to blend about three-quarters of the soup; it should be creamy with some whole chunks of potatoes. If you don't have a immersion blender, then transfer about three-quarters of the soup to a blender and puree, lifting the lid after a moment to let the steam escape, then add it back to the soup.

Mix in the chard. Let the soup simmer for about 5 minutes, until the chard is soft. Mix in the tempeh, taste for salt, and serve.

PREPARE THE TEMPEH:

In a sauté pan, crumble the tempeh and add enough water to almost cover it. Cover the pan and, over high heat, steam the tempeh until most of the water is absorbed, about 10 minutes. Drain the remaining water and add the rest of the ingredients. Cook over medium heat, stirring occasionally, until lightly browned, about 10 minutes. Set aside until ready to add to the soup.

Manhattan Glam Chowder

SERVES 4 • ACTIVE TIME: 15 MINUTES • TOTAL TIME: 40 MINUTES

Boston and New York will catfight over almost anything—not just baseball but soup, too. Manhattan clam chowder is tomato based, rather than cream based as they do in New England. I grew up slurping bowlfuls of this soup whenever it was on the diner menu, not out of NYC patriotism but because it was irresistibly delicious. I was never a big fan of seafood, but the mellow ocean flavor of nori is just right and not at all overpowering. In Glam Chowder the clams are left alone and a few shiitake mushrooms stand in, giving the soup that expected occasional chewiness. Garnish with a crumbled saltine-type cracker for authenticity.

2 teaspoons olive oil
1 small onion, diced small
2 ribs celery, sliced thinly
3 cloves garlic, minced
   Several pinches of freshly ground black pepper
½ teaspoon salt
¼ pound shiitake mushrooms, sliced ½ inch thick
2 bay leaves
2 teaspoons dried thyme
2 sheets nori
1 pound Yukon Gold potatoes, cut into ½-inch chunks
1 (15-ounce) can diced tomatoes
2 cups vegetable broth
1 teaspoon agave nectar

Preheat a 4-quart pot over medium-high heat. Sauté the onions and celery in the oil until the onions are translucent, about 5 minutes. Use a little nonstick cooking spray or broth if needed. Add the garlic, pepper, and salt, and sauté for another minute.

Mix in the mushrooms, bay leaves, and thyme. Use your fingers to crush the nori sheets right into the soup. It should be in small confetti pieces and rain down into the pot as if it's New Year's Eve (see tip). Sauté for about 3 minutes to get the mushrooms tender and to toast the nori just a bit.

Add the potatoes, tomatoes, and vegetable broth. Cover the pot and bring to a boil. Once boiling, lower heat to a simmer and cook for 15 to 20 minutes, until the potatoes are tender.

Add the agave and taste for salt and seasoning. Ladle into bowls and garnish each with a cracker, if desired.

∿ NUTRITION TIP

Despite widespread claims, seaweed is never a source of vitamin B12. Occasionally it shows up on the package because it contains a B12 analog that is similar enough that the tests cannot differentiate. ↵

∿ INGREDIENT SCAVENGER HUNT

You're probably already familiar with nori; it's the type of seaweed wrapper used for rolling sushi. It feels a bit like paper, which isn't surprising because it goes through a similar compression process. In this soup, the nori is used more as an herb would be. Not all noris are created equal—the texture of the different brands may vary, so if you're not able to shred the nori with your hands, then just roll it up and chop it on the cutting board, then add to the soup. Nori is fairly easy to find these days, as most supermarkets have a Japanese section, or at least an Asian section. Once the package is opened, store the remainder in a sealed plastic bag in your pantry to keep fresh. ↵

Yam & Black Bean Soup with Orange & Cilantro

SERVES 8 • ACTIVE TIME: 20 MINUTES • TOTAL TIME: 45 MINUTES

PER SERVING
(⅛ RECIPE):
Calories: 240
Calories from fat: 15
Total fat: 2 g
Saturated fat: 0 g
Trans fat: 0 g
Total carb: 50 g
Fiber: 9 g
Sugars: 11 g
Protein: 7 g
Cholesterol: 0 mg
Sodium: 560 mg
Vitamin A: 490%
Vitamin C: 50%
Calcium: 8%
Iron: 15%

A little orange juice elevates the flavor of the yams in this flirty soup (can soup be flirty?) studded with black beans and spiked with a little heat from serrano peppers. Fresh squeezed orange juice is preferred, but you can use the not-from-concentrate kind, too.

2 teaspoons olive oil

1 red onion, sliced thinly

2 serrano peppers, seeded and minced

2 cloves garlic, minced

4 plum tomatoes, chopped

2 teaspoons ground cumin

1½ teaspoons salt

3 pounds yams, peeled and cut into roughly ¾-inch chunks

3 cups water

1 cup orange juice

1½ cups cooked black beans, or 1 (16-ounce) can, drained and rinsed

½ cup fresh cilantro leaves and stems, chopped
Extra cilantro, for garnish

Preheat a 4-quart pot over medium heat. Sauté the onions in the olive oil for about 5 minutes, until softened. Add the serrano pepper and garlic, and sauté for another minute. Add the tomatoes, cumin, and salt. Turn up the heat a bit and cook the tomatoes down for about 5 minutes. Add the yams and water. Cover and bring to a boil.

Once boiling, turn down the heat to simmer and leave the cover slightly ajar so that steam can escape. Simmer for about 15 minutes; the yams should be pierced easily with a fork.

Turn off the heat. Use a potato masher to mash the yams five or six times, leaving some whole. Add the orange juice, beans, and cilantro. Let sit for about 10 minutes; the beans should be heated through. Stir well and serve garnished with cilantro.

Summer Lovin' Curried Corn & Veggie Chowder

SERVES 4 • ACTIVE TIME: 20 MINUTES • TOTAL TIME: 45 MINUTES

This is a fabulous way to spend a summer night when corn and zucchini are plentiful and the kitchen has cooled down enough to turn on the stove. But you know, if the mood strikes in winter, don't let the title dissuade you. You'd think that this chowder was just swimming in oil and fat, but it's actually really nice and light. A little coconut milk and arrowroot help out with the thickening, and pureeing the corn helps out with the creaminess. I like it hot, so I use a ½ teaspoon of red pepper flakes. If you prefer a mild curry, just leave it out or use ¼ teaspoon instead. And if you'd like to serve it with something, I think a cup of simple brown basmati rice would be just loverly.

1 teaspoon canola oil
1 cup shallots, chopped finely
1 red bell pepper, seeded and chopped finely
4 cloves garlic, minced
1 tablespoon minced fresh ginger
½ teaspoon red pepper flakes (optional)
1 zucchini, sliced into small pieces (about ½ pound)
1¾ cups corn, from 3 ears corn (reserve cobs)
½ teaspoon salt
3 cups vegetable broth
2 teaspoons arrowroot powder
½ cup peeled, finely chopped carrots (I cheat and use baby carrots, 'cause the work is half done for you)
1 heaping tablespoon mild curry powder
¾ cup light coconut milk
Juice of ½ lime, or to taste
Fresh cilantro, for garnish (optional)

PER SERVING (¼ RECIPE):
Calories: 180
Calories from fat: 50
Total fat: 5 g
Saturated fat: 2.5 g
Trans fat: 0 g
Total carb: 30 g
Fiber: 4 g
Sugars: 8 g
Protein: 7 g
Cholesterol: 0 mg
Sodium: 760 mg
Vitamin A: 80%
Vitamin C: 100%
Calcium: 6%
Iron: 15%

Preheat a 4-quart pot over medium-high heat. Sauté the shallots and red bell pepper in the oil until translucent, about 4 minutes. Use a little non-stick cooking spray or broth if needed. Add the garlic, ginger, and red pepper flakes, and sauté for another minute. Add the zucchini and corn and sprinkle in the salt. Cook for about 3 minutes, stirring once.

Measure 1 cup of the broth into a measuring cup. Mix in the arrowroot with a fork until dissolved. You do this because it's just easier to get the arrowroot dissolved into smaller quantities of liquid. Add the arrowroot mixture to the pot, along with the rest of the broth. Mix in the carrots and curry powder. Cover the pot and bring to a boil. Once boiling, break the corn cobs in half and add them to the pot. Lower the heat to a simmer and cook for about 20 minutes, or until the vegetables are tender. Remove the corn cobs. Add the coconut milk and lime juice.

> ❧ TIP This recipe uses a method that really makes corn chowder shine: Let the corn cobs stew in the pot. They hold lots of maize-y flavor, so don't let 'em go to waste. At the end, you remove the cobs and only your delicious soup knows they were ever there. I suppose you can use frozen corn instead, but only if you're really crunched for time. ☙

Use an immersion blender to blend about half of the soup. If you don't have an immersion blender (get one!), then transfer about half of the soup to a blender or food processor and puree until smooth, then add back to the pot. If the soup is still steaming hot, make sure to either keep the opening on top of your food processor open, or lift the lid often for steam to escape. If steam builds up in a closed container it can explode the lid off. Ouch.

Taste for seasoning. Serve garnished with cilantro, if you like.

Red Lentil & Root Veggie Dal

SERVES 6 • ACTIVE TIME: 20 MINUTES • TOTAL TIME: 45 MINUTES

Root vegetables perk up this characteristically humble dish. Dal is a velvety, spicy stew served throughout India and some parts of the Middle East, made from any quick cooking "split" legume. Here, we use red lentils and simplify spices a bit to make for an easy and pantry-friendly soup. The root veggies add a creamy texture and an earthy peppery taste that is just slightly sweet. I use parsnip and rutabaga for this soup, but you can use which ever root veggies you like. Serve over brown basmati rice.

2	teaspoons olive oil
1	medium-size onion, diced finely
3	cloves garlic, minced
1	tablespoon minced fresh ginger
¼	teaspoon red pepper flakes
2	teaspoons coriander seeds, crushed
2 to 3	teaspoons mild curry powder (start with 2 teaspoons and add more at the end, if you like)
1	teaspoon ground cumin
¼	teaspoon ground cardamom
¼	teaspoon ground cinnamon
1¼	teaspoons salt
4	cups vegetable broth
1	cup dried red lentils
¾	pound parsnip, peeled and diced into ½-inch pieces (about 2 cups)
¾	pound rutabaga or turnip, peeled and diced into ½-inch pieces (about 2 cups)
1	cup baby carrots, cut into ½-inch pieces
	Lime slices, for serving (optional)

**PER SERVING
(⅙ RECIPE):**
Calories: 240
Calories from fat: 20
Total fat: 2.5 g
Saturated fat: 0 g
Trans fat: 0 g
Total carb: 44 g
Fiber: 16 g
Sugars: 12 g
Protein: 12 g
Cholesterol: 0 mg
Sodium: 980 mg
Vitamin A: 100%
Vitamin C: 50%
Calcium: 10%
Iron: 20%

Preheat a 4-quart pot over medium-high heat. Sauté the onions in the oil until translucent, about 4 minutes. Add the garlic, ginger, and red pepper flakes, and sauté for another minute.

Add the remaining spices and salt, and sauté for about 30 seconds, then add the broth, lentils, and the remaining vegetables. Cover the pot and bring to a boil, keeping a close eye on it. Once it's boiling, lower the heat to a simmer and cook for about 20 minutes, until the lentils are creamy and the vegetables are soft. If neccesary, thin the soup by adding up to a cup of water. Taste for salt and seasonings.

Let the soup sit for 10 minutes or so for maximum flavor. Serve garnished with lime slices.

> ∽ TIP To peel a rutabaga or turnip, hold it stem side up and use your 8-inch chef's knife to thinly slice off the peel, running the knife down the side of the vegetable from top to bottom. The more practice you get, the easier it will be; you just have to know where the curve is to get it as thin as possible. ∾

> ∽ TIP As the years go by, my coriander seed–crushing techniques get more and more refined. The easiest way to crush coriander is to place the seeds in a plastic sandwich bag and roll them with a rolling pin for about a minute. I keep a plastic bag in my spice cabinet for this very reason, and just reuse it as much as I can until it falls apart. It's really a great method to coax the most flavor out of your coriander. If you really, really don't feel like it, 1½ teaspoons of ground coriander can be used in its place. ∾

Peruvian Purple Potato Soup

SERVES 6 • ACTIVE TIME: 15 MINUTES • TOTAL TIME: 45 MINUTES

Why is this soup Peruvian? Maybe because purple potatoes are native to Peru, or maybe because I love alliteration. When I spot purple potatoes at the farmers' market, I can't stop myself from lugging home a ton of them. Slice them open and they're such a gorgeous hue, the kind of purple you want to paint your room on a Saturday evening when you're fifteen and have no Cure concert to go to. But these days you don't have to go to the farmers' market to procure some of these beauties; many well-stocked supermarkets sell purple potatoes, or at least blue potatoes, which would be great in this soup, too. After boiling the potatoes the color does fade just a tad, so I cheat and grate in some beet at the end. Unless you're a food photographer or entering the soup into a purple food competition, that probably isn't exactly necessary.

PER SERVING
(⅙ RECIPE):
Calories: 150
Calories from fat: 10
Total fat: 1 g
Saturated fat: 0 g
Trans fat: 0 g
Total carb: 30 g
Fiber: 4 g
Sugars: 4 g
Protein: 5 g
Cholesterol: 0 mg
Sodium: 570 mg
Vitamin A: 0%
Vitamin C: 60%
Calcium: 4%
Iron: 8%

1 teaspoon olive oil
1 small yellow onion, chopped finely
2 jalapeños, seeded and sliced
2 bay leaves
3 cloves garlic, minced
4 cups vegetable broth
2 pounds purple potatoes, peeled and cut into ¾-inch chunks
½ teaspoon salt, plus more to taste
¼ cup lightly packed fresh cilantro, chopped
1 tablespoon freshly squeezed lime juice, or to taste
A little grated beet, for color (optional)

Preheat a 4-quart pot over medium heat. Sauté the onions, jalapeños, and bay leaves for about 7 minutes, until translucent. Add the garlic and sauté for 3 minutes more.

Add the potatoes, water, and salt. Cover and bring to a boil. Once boiling, lower the heat a bit to a slow simmer and cook until the potatoes are tender, 15 to 18 minutes.

Use an immersion blender to puree half the soup, or transfer half of the soup to a blender or food processor and puree. Be sure to let the steam escape between pulses so that it doesn't build up and explode all over you. If using a blender, return the pureed soup to the pot and mix.

Add the cilantro and lime, and taste for salt. Grate in a little bit of beet, using a Microplane grater if you've got one. Use about a tablespoon. Let the soup sit for at least 5 minutes for the flavors to blend. Serve!

> ∾ TIP *Peel the potatoes while the onions are sautéeing, or if you don't care about a little potato skin in your soup, live on the edge and forgo the peeling altogether.* ∾

Smoky Split Pea Soup

SERVES 6 • ACTIVE TIME: 15 MINUTES • TOTAL TIME: 1 HOUR

What kind of soup chapter would this be if there were no split pea recipe? I'd be the laughingstock (no pun intended) of the soup community. This is what you wanna slurp on any day of the week, for any and every occasion. This version is made smoky and sultry with a dose of smoked paprika.

- 1 teaspoon olive oil
- 1 medium-size onion, diced small
- 4 cloves garlic, minced
  Several pinches of freshly ground black pepper
- 1 teaspoon salt
- 4 teaspoons smoked paprika
- 2 teaspoons dried thyme
- 1½ cups diced carrots
- 1¼ cups split peas
- 6 cups vegetable broth
- 1 tablespoon freshly squeezed lemon juice, or to taste

Preheat a 4-quart pot over medium-high heat. Sauté the onions in the oil until translucent, about 4 minutes. Add the garlic, pepper, and salt, and sauté for another minute. Add the paprika and thyme, and stir continuously for about 15 seconds to toast the spices a bit.

Add the carrots, split peas, and broth. Cover the pot and bring to a boil, keeping a close eye on it. Once it's boiling, lower the heat to a simmer and cook for about 40 minutes, until the lentils are creamy. Stir occasionally to prevent the soup from burning at the bottom. If necessary, thin the soup with water. Add the lemon juice and taste for salt and seasonings.

Let the soup sit for 10 minutes or so for maximum flavor and serve.

CHAPTER 8

Comfort Curries, Chili, & Stews

THIS CHAPTER IS ALL ABOUT THE COMFORT: SAUCY, SAVORY, and filling one-pot meals that come together in a snap. Aromatic curries, spicy chili, and hearty stews, these are weeknight meals that hit the spot. These dishes are also a great opportunity to flex your spice rack muscles. Build your spice arsenal as you build your repertoire, recipe by recipe. Take advantage of the bulk bins at your health food store or Indian market; this way the spices are not only cheaper, but you can buy smaller quantities. You'll never have to let spices expire or collect dust because you'll be buying in manageable quantities that you know you'll use.

It's also a great time to experiment with new ingredients. I utilize every bean under the sun, leave no grain unturned and no veggie left behind, to bring satisfying meals with variety to your stovetop.

Many of these recipes come together in 30 minutes, and the ones that take longer don't require more work, just a bit more time. But don't let longer cooking times deter you; it just means you've got more downtime to plan the week's menu or study for the bar or play Rock Band. You know, whatever you feel like doing.

Most of the recipes call for a four-quart pot. A heavy-bottomed, stainless-steel pot with a secure lid and a long handle is my weapon of choice. Definitely invest in something sturdy. That beat-up piece of aluminum from the dollar store just won't cut it.

Above all, have fun with this chapter. Try the recipes out as written if you're new at this, but don't be afraid to experiment with what's in season and what you have on hand. That's what comfort's all about: knowing things will be okay, no matter what.

2nd Avenue Vegetable Korma

SERVES 4 • ACTIVE TIME: 20 MINUTES • TOTAL TIME: 30 MINUTES

PER SERVING
(¼ RECIPE):
Calories: 180
Calories from fat: 45
Total fat: 5 g
Saturated fat: 2.5 g
Trans fat: 0 g
Total carb: 29 g
Fiber: 9 g
Sugars: 12 g
Protein: 9 g
Cholesterol: 0 mg
Sodium: 720 mg
Vitamin A: 210%
Vitamin C: 180%
Calcium: 10%
Iron: 15%

One of my favorite restaurants in NYC is Madras, located downtown on Second Avenue. Rumor has it that they are closing, and maybe by the time you read this they will be gone. It's too bad because they serve the best vegan southern Indian food I've ever had, and this vegetable korma is a tribute. Vegetable korma is generally a rich and creamy curry with braised vegetables. Their version has a lot of coconut milk; mine has a bit of light coconut milk, but it's still rich and yummy and it takes only 30 minutes. So if you can get to Sixth Street and Second Avenue in 30 minutes, then godspeed. If not, then try this dish over some brown basmati rice. It would also be delicious over mashed sweet potato or the **Cranberry-Cashew Biryani** (page 67).

1 teaspoon olive oil
1 small red onion, quartered and sliced thinly
3 cloves garlic, minced
2 tablespoons minced fresh ginger
2 teaspoons curry powder
1 teaspoon garam masala
1 teaspoon ground cumin
½ teaspoon ground coriander
½ teaspoon salt
2 cups vegetable broth
1½ pounds cauliflower, trimmed and cut into florets
1 pound zucchini, cut on a bias in ¼-inch slices
½ pound carrots, peeled and cut on a bias in ¼-inch slices
¾ cup frozen peas
¾ cup light coconut milk
1 teaspoon agave nectar
½ cup chopped fresh cilantro (optional)
  Extra chopped fresh cilantro, for garnish

Preheat a 4-quart pot over medium heat. Sauté the onion in the oil for about 5 minutes, until translucent. Use a little nonstick cooking spray if needed. Add the garlic and ginger, and sauté for another minute.

Add the broth to deglaze the pan. Mix in the spices and salt. Add the cauliflower, zucchini, and carrots. They won't be competely submerged, but that's okay. Cover the pot and turn up the heat to bring the broth to a boil. Let boil for 7 to 10 minutes, until the veggies are tender.

Add the peas, coconut milk, agave, and cilantro (if using). Taste for salt. Turn off the heat and let the flavors meld for about 5 minutes. Serve the korma in bowls over rice, garnished with cilantro.

> ∾ TIP *Get colorful! Combine the zucchini with yellow summer squash and switch out half of the cauliflower with broccoli.* ∾

> ∾ TIP *If you'd like to add some protein to this dish, try a cup and a half of chickpeas, or some dry-fried tofu (see the* **Hoison–Mustard Tofu** *recipe, page 153). Add either along with the peas and stuff at the end, just enough to heat through.* ∾

Curried Chickpeas & Greens

SERVES 6 • ACTIVE TIME: 30 MINUTES • TOTAL TIME: 20 MINUTES

PER SERVING
(⅙ RECIPE):
Calories: 240
Calories from fat: 50
Total fat: 5 g
Saturated fat: 0 g
Trans fat: 0 g
Total carb: 41 g
Fiber: 10 g
Sugars: 9 g
Protein: 13 g
Cholesterol: 0 mg
Sodium: 670 mg
Vitamin A: 470%
Vitamin C: 320%
Calcium: 30%
Iron: 30%

When my best friend and I first went vegetarian in the '80s, we spent a bunch of time living on cheeseless pizza and broccoli from a Chinese takeout place. My best friend's dad was Pakistani, and when he heard what we were eating, he insisted we visit one of the Pakistani restaurants on Coney Island Avenue in Brooklyn. And my love of Chana Saag, whose name means "chickpeas and greens," was born. I've been making this recipe in some form or other for about twenty years, and I still can't get enough of it. Leafy greens are cooked down until tender and velvety, punctuated by chickpeas and underlined with spice. Serve with brown basmati rice, or with any of the Indian-style sides.

2 teaspoons olive oil
2 teaspoons mustard seeds
1 small onion, diced small
4 cloves garlic, minced
2 tablespoons minced fresh ginger
½ teaspoon red pepper flakes (optional, if you like it spicy)
1 tablespoon curry powder
2 teaspoons ground cumin
1 teaspoon ground coriander
1 teaspoon garam masala
1 teaspoon salt
1 (12-ounce can) crushed tomatoes
2 pounds kale, coarse stems removed, chopped finely
1 (28-ounce) can chickpeas, drained and rinsed

Preheat a 4-quart pot over medium heat. Pour 1 teaspoon of the oil into the pot and use a spatula to coat the bottom. Add the mustard seeds. Cover the pot and let the seeds pop for about a minute, or until the popping slows down, mixing once. If the seeds don't pop, turn up the heat a bit until they do. Add the other teaspoon of oil and sauté the onion for

4 to 7 minutes, until translucent. Use a little nonstick cooking spray if needed. Add the garlic, ginger, and red pepper flakes, and sauté for another minute. Add the tomatoes and mix to deglaze the pot. Let cook for about 3 minutes, then add the curry, cumin, coriander, garam masala, and salt, and mix well.

Add the kale in batches, mixing well after each addition. It may seem like way too much, but it will cook down. Cover the pot, let simmer for a minute, lift the lid, and stir. After doing this three times or so, the kale should be well cooked down. Simmer and cook covered for 10 minutes, stirring occasionally. The greens should be very tender.

Add the chickpeas and cook for another 5 minutes or so. Taste for salt and serve.

> ∾ NOTE I remember when it cost $1.50 for the chickpeas, a side of rice, and a piece of naan bread. Even in the '80s that was quite a deal! We would wrap everything up in the naan so we could walk down the street with it, because in Brooklyn, you walk down the street eating (see Saturday Night Fever opening sequence). You can use a whole wheat wrap for roughly the same effect. ∾

Variation

If you like Saag Paneer (paneer being a firm, cubed cheese), then try this dish with tofu instead. Use the dry-fry method for cubed tofu (see the **Hoisin-Mustard Tofu** recipe, page 153), and add it in place of the chickpeas.

> ∾ NUTRITION TIP Kale is not known for its fat content—a 1-ounce serving has 0.4 grams, which is rounded down to zero. But when eaten in large portions, this adds up—in a good way! Kale is a source of omega-3 fatty acids and its omega-6 to omega-3 ratio is fantastic, up there with flaxseeds. When one eats many servings a week of such dark leafy greens as kale, it can be considered a good source of omega-3. ∾

Eggplant–Chickpea Curry

SERVES 6 • ACTIVE TIME: 20 MINUTES • TOTAL TIME: 1½ HOURS

This well-cooked eggplant is so rich, silky, and full bodied that you will never guess that it has only a teaspoon of oil. In fact, don't tell anyone, because with each flavorful forkful they'll believe you less and less until they never trust you again.

In this dish I've made use of the old standby, curry powder, as well as garam masala, which has an aromatic blend of coriander, clove, and cardamom. The cooking time is a bit long, but the dish is pretty easy, so even if you've never cooked eggplant before don't be intimidated; this recipe would make a great introduction. I've always noticed that eggplant will be super stubborn at first and then suddenly and rapidly decide to comply, so if your eggplant hasn't broken down in 20 minutes or so, up the heat a bit and check again soon. Serve over brown jasmine or basmati rice, or try the **Cranberry–Cashew Biryani** (page 67).

1 teaspoon oil
1 small white onion, chopped finely
3 cloves garlic, minced
1 tablespoon minced fresh ginger
¼ teaspoon red pepper flakes (optional, use if you like it spicy)
1 pound tomatoes, chopped roughly (3 average-size; about 2 cups)
2 pounds eggplant, cut into ¾-inch cubes
1 teaspoon salt
2 teaspoons mild curry powder
2 teaspoons garam masala
1 teaspoon ground cumin
1 cup vegetable broth
1 (15-ounce can) chickpeas, drained and rinsed (about 1½ cups)
Chopped fresh cilantro, for garnish (optional)

Preheat a 4-quart pot over medium heat. Sauté the onion in the oil for about 5 minutes, until translucent. Use a little nonstick cooking spray if needed. Add the garlic, ginger, and red pepper flakes (if using), and sauté for another minute. Mix in the tomato, eggplant, and salt, and cook, stirring constantly, for about a minute. The tomato should deglaze the pan.

Mix in the curry powder, garam masala, and ground cumin. Add the vegetable broth, stir, and cover the pot. Bring the mixture to a slow boil and cook with the pot covered for about 40 minutes, stirring occasionally. The eggplant should be mostly broken down by this point. Add the chickpeas and cook uncovered for another 10 minutes, stirring for about a minute at first (to further break down the eggplant) and then occasionally.

Taste for salt and serve garnished with cilantro.

Potato-Spinach Curry

SERVES 6 • ACTIVE TIME: 20 MINUTES • TOTAL TIME: 45 MINUTES

Inspired by the Indian dish Saag Aloo but with a million shortcuts, this curry hits the spot when I'm craving velvety mushy spinach, which is more often than you'd think. I really love frozen spinach here because if you were going to use the equivalent amount in fresh it would be a lot more work, a lot more expensive, and it just wouldn't get as creamy. But try your best to find the kind that is clearly marked "chopped" as opposed to plain old frozen spinach.

The potatoes give the dish extra creaminess plus the added bonus of . . . potatoes! It's also a fun recipe because you get to pop the mustard seeds at the beginning. Serve this curry over brown jasmine or basmati rice, or the **Tamarind Quinoa** (page 84). For some extra protein, top with a few slices **Masala Baked Tofu** (page 146).

2 teaspoons vegetable oil
1 tablespoon yellow mustard seeds
1 small onion, diced small
4 cloves garlic, minced
2 tablespoons minced fresh ginger
¼ teaspoon red pepper flakes
2 plum tomatoes, chopped
1 tablespoon curry powder
1 teaspoon ground cumin
½ teaspoon salt
2 cups vegetable broth
2 pounds Yukon Gold potatoes, cut into ½-inch chunks
1 pound chopped frozen spinach
1 tablespoon freshly squeezed lime juice

Preheat a 4-quart pot over medium heat. Pour 1 teaspoon of the oil into the pot and use a spatula to help it coat the bottom. Add the mustard seeds. Cover the pot and let the seeds pop for about a minute, or until the popping slows down, mixing once. If the seeds don't pop, turn up the heat a bit until they do. Add the other teaspoon of oil and sauté the onion for about 5 minutes, until translucent. Use a little nonstick cooking spray if needed. Add the garlic, ginger, and red pepper flakes, and sauté for another minute. Add the tomato and mix to deglaze the pot. Let cook for about 3 minutes, then add the curry, cumin, and salt, and mix well.

> **TIP** *If you can't find Yukon Gold potatoes, just use red potatoes or the thinnest-skinned potatoes you can find. That way, no peeling necessary!*

Add the potatoes and vegetable broth. The potatoes may be peeking out of the top of the broth, and that's okay. Turn up the heat, cover the pot, and bring the mixture to a boil. Once boiling, lower the heat to a simmer and cook, covered, for 15 minutes, stirring occasionally.

Add the spinach and mix well. Cover and cook for 5 more minutes, or until the spinach has thawed. Mix well and cook for another 10 minutes, or until the spinach is good and mushy and the potatoes are tender. Add the lime juice, taste for salt, and serve.

Thai Roasted Root Vegetable Curry

SERVES 6 • ACTIVE TIME: 30 MINUTES • TOTAL TIME: 45 MINUTES

(CAN BE MADE GLUTEN FREE IF USING GF TAMARI IN PLACE OF CURRY PASTE AND SOY SAUCE)

~~~~~~~~~~
PER SERVING
(⅙ RECIPE):
Calories: 210
Calories from fat: 30
Total fat: 3.5 g
Saturated fat: 1.5 g
Trans fat: 0 g
Total carb: 42 g
Fiber: 11 g
Sugars: 17 g
Protein: 7 g
Cholesterol: 0 mg
Sodium: 790 mg
Vitamin A: 170%
Vitamin C: 170%
Calcium: 15%
Iron: 15%

Ever wonder what Thanksgiving at a Thai restaurant might taste like? Earthy, roasty root veggies and Brussels sprouts join forces with aromatic and sweet coconut Thai curry, in an unexpected flavor combination that ends up making so much sense! Serve with brown basmati rice.

1	pound rutabagas, peeled and cut into ¾-inch chunks
1	pound parsnips, peeled and cut into ¾-inch chunks
1	pound Brussels sprouts, cut in half lenghtwise
2 to 3	tablespoons green curry paste
	Small red onion, cut into thinly sliced half-moons
2	cloves garlic, minced
1	tablespoon minced fresh ginger
1	cup baby carrots, sliced in half diagonally
1	cup peeled, small-diced sweet potato
3	cups vegetable broth
1	tablespoon soy sauce
¾	cup light coconut milk
2	tablespoons freshly squeezed lime juice
1	tablespoons light agave nectar
1	cup fresh cilantro, for garnish

First, let's roast the veggies. Preheat the oven to 425°F. Line two baking sheets with parchment paper. Put the rutabagas, parsnips, and Brussel sprouts in a single layer on the baking sheets and spray lightly with non-stick cooking spray. Roast for about 30 minutes, tossing once and spraying with a little more cooking spray. The rutabaga should be pierced easily with a fork. Remove from the oven and set aside until ready to use.

Meanwhile, prepare the curry. Preheat a 4-quart pot over medium high heat. Place 2 tablespoons of the curry paste in the pot and mix in the onions. Sauté for about 2 minutes. Add a splash of water if it seems to be sticking excessively. Add the garlic and ginger, and sauté for another 2 minutes. Add the carrots, sweet potato, broth, and soy sauce, cover, and bring to a slow rolling boil. Cook until the sweet potato is not just tender but mushy, about 20 minutes. It should be mushy enough to thicken up the stew when mashed with a fork. Go ahead and lightly mash it.

Add the coconut milk, lime juice, and agave to the pot and mix. Taste for salt and spice. You may want to add up to another tablespoon of curry paste, depending on the strength of the brand you used.

Add the roasted veggies and serve with chopped cilantro as a garnish.

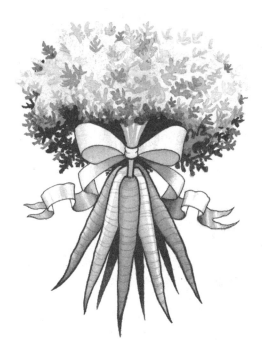

Classic Black Bean & Veggie Chili

SERVES 6 • ACTIVE TIME: 20 MINUTES • TOTAL TIME: 40 MINUTES

As the name suggests, this is it, that classic chili that seems to be a staple vegetarian option at diners nationwide: chili with black beans, corn, zucchini, and carrots. There are no bells and whistles here, just a good, dependable chili recipe with plenty of flexibility for whatever veggies you might have on hand. For best results, skip that ninety-nine-cent chili powder and use a high-quality one; it still won't be very expensive. Serve the chili with rice or corn bread.

1	teaspoon olive oil
1	onion, diced small
1	green bell pepper, seeded and diced small
3	cloves garlic, minced
1	large carrot, diced small
1	pound zucchini, cut into medium dice
1	cup corn, fresh or frozen (thaw first if frozen)
1½	cups vegetable broth
3	tablespoons chili powder
2	teaspoons ground cumin
1	teaspoon dried oregano
1	teaspoon salt
	Several pinches of freshly ground black pepper
1	(28-ounce) can diced tomatoes
2	tablespoons tomato paste
1	(15-ounce can) black beans, drained and rinsed
1	cup lightly packed fresh cilantro, chopped
2	teaspoons agave nectar
2	tablespoons freshly squeezed lime juice

Preheat a 4-quart pot over medium-high heat. Sauté the onions and bell pepper in oil until translucent, 4 to 7 minutes. Add the garlic and sauté for another minute, using nonstick cooking spray or a splash of water if it's sticking.

Mix in the carrot, zucchini, and corn. Add the vegetable broth, chili powder, cumin, oregano, salt, and black pepper. The veggies should be mostly submerged, but it's okay if some are poking out; they will cook down.

Cover the pot and bring to a boil, keeping a close eye on it. Once boiling, lower the heat to a simmer and cook for about 10 minutes, until the carrots are fairly tender and the zucchini is soft. Add the tomatoes, tomato paste, black beans, and cilantro, cover, and cook for about 10 more minutes. Mix in the agave and lime juice. Taste for salt and seasoning, and serve.

> ᗑ NUTRITION TIP *Foodies turn their noses up at frozen vegetables, but the methods for freezing vegetables have come a long way and frozen can have even more nutrients than fresh! How? The vegetables are flash-frozen soon after being harvested and the nutrients are retained. Those "fresh" vegetables in the bottom of the fridge that you have been meaning to eat have lost more nutrients over time. Yes, fresh is better, if used while fresh, but don't shy away from the convenience of frozen. You're still getting all that nutrition!* ᗑ

Chipotle Chili with Sweet Potatoes & Brussels Sprouts

SERVES 6 • ACTIVE TIME: 20 MINUTES • TOTAL TIME: 45 MINUTES

This was one of those "clean out my cupboard and fridge" recipes. I had plenty of sweet potatoes and Brussels sprouts left over from holiday festivities and this was a flavorful and filling way to use them up. I put the recipe up on my blog and it went viral! No, not really, but lots of people made it and loved it so I had to include it in the book. Robust Brussels sprouts complement the sweetness of the sweet potatoes nicely, and the smokiness of the chipotle provides a perfect backdrop.

  1 teaspoon olive oil

  1 red onion, diced small

  4 cloves garlic, minced

  1 tablespoon coriander seeds, crushed

  2 teaspoons dried oregano

  3 chipotles in adobo, seeded and chopped

1½ pounds sweet potatoes (2 average-size), peeled and cut into ¾-inch pieces

12 ounces Brussels sprouts, quartered lengthwise (about 2 cups)

  2 teaspoons ground cumin

  1 tablespoon chili powder

  1 (28-ounce) can crushed tomatoes

  1 cup water

  1 (16-ounce) can pinto beans, drained and rinsed (about 1½ cups)

1½ teaspoons salt

    Freshly squeezed lime juice

In a 4-quart pot over medium heat, sauté the onion in the olive oil for 5 to 7 minutes, until translucent. Add the garlic, coriander seeds, and oregano, and sauté for a minute more. Add the remaining ingredients (except the lime juice). Mix well. The sweet potatoes and Brussel sprouts will be peeking out of the tomato sauce, but don't worry, they will cook down.

Cover the pot and bring it to a boil, then lower the heat to simmer and cook for about half an hour, stirring often, until the sweet potatoes are tender but not mushy. Squeeze in the lime juice to taste and adjust any other seasonings. Let the chili sit uncovered for at least 10 minutes before eating.

∾ INGREDIENT SCAVENGER HUNT

The chipotle has got to be this century's sun-dried tomato. Barely glance at a menu and you'll catch it weaseling its way into soups, sauces, omelets, even desserts. But the chipotle's pervasive stature is not unearned. Its smoky heat adds so much flavor to anything it touches, you'd be hard pressed not to reach for it when you want to whip up something fast and tasty.

Watch any cooking show in the last decade and they'll be sure to tell you that a chipotle is a smoked jalapeño. You can find them dried, but more commonly they come stewed in a can with adobo, a vinegary tomato-based sauce. I usually remove the seeds before using; that way you can get more chipotle flavor without adding too much heat. Because you won't be using an entire can for a recipe, store the rest in a plastic bag and freeze. Just thaw when you need it again. ∾

Chili Verde con Papas

SERVES 6 • ACTIVE TIME: 20 MINUTES • TOTAL TIME: 45 MINUTES

If you're looking for a chili change of pace, then go green! Tomatillos are like little presents already wrapped in nature's gift wrapping. Just remove those papery husks and you have a tart, juicy green tomato just perfect for stewing up in a spicy chili. This makes a great one-pot meal: you've got kale for your veggie, potatoes for carbs, and beans for protein. But if you want to serve it over some rice or with corn bread, I'm not going to stop you.

- 1 pound baby Yukon Gold potatoes or other thin-skinned creamy potato, cut into ½-inch pieces
- 1 teaspoon vegetable oil
- 1 large yellow onion, diced small
- 3 jalapeños, seeded and sliced thinly
- 1 green bell pepper, seeded and cut into medium dice
- 4 cloves garlic, minced
- 1 tablespoon ground cumin
- 1 teaspoon dried oregano (Mexican oregano, preferably)
- 1 teaspoon salt
- ⅓ cup dry white wine
- 1 pound tomatillos (about 10 small to medium ones), papery skin removed, washed and chopped into ½- to ¾-inch pieces
- 1 pound kale, coarse stems removed, chopped into bite-size pieces
- 2 cups vegetable broth
- 1 cup loosely packed fresh cilantro
- ¼ cup chopped scallions, plus extra for garnish
- 1½ cups navy beans
  Juice of 1 lime
- 1 teaspoon light agave nectar

Place the chopped potatoes in a small saucepan, cover with water, and bring to a boil. Let boil, covered, for a little less than 20 minutes, until the potatoes are pierced easily with a fork). Drain and set aside. Prepare everything else while the potatoes are boiling.

Preheat a 4-quart pot over medium-high heat. Sauté the onion, jalapeños, and green pepper in the oil for about 7 minutes, until everything is softened and the onions are slightly browned. Use a little nonstick cooking spray and a splash of water if things appear dry.

Add the garlic, cumin, oregano, and salt. Sauté for a minute more, until the garlic is fragrant.

Add the white wine and tomatillos, turn up the heat a bit, and let the wine reduce and the tomatillos release their juices, about 5 minutes.

Add the vegetable broth, scallions, and ½ cup of the cilantro. Turn down the heat to a simmer (medium-low), cover, and cook for about 5 minutes, just to heat through.

Use an immersion blender to partially puree everything. If you don't have one, then transfer half the mixture to a food processor and blend smooth, then transfer back to the pot. Don't forget that if you are using a blender you need to be careful not to have a steam explosion, so pulse quickly and then lift the lid to let steam escape, then pulse again and repeat.

Add the kale, cover, and cook for about 10 minutes, until the kale is soft. Taste for sweetness/tartness. Add the cooked potatoes and the beans, and simmer for a few more minutes, until everything is heated through. Add the remaining cilantro, lime juice to taste, and agave. Taste for tartness and sweetness and adjust as needed. Ladle into bowls and garnish with the cilantro and scallions.

Lentil & Eggplant Chili Mole

MAKES 6 SERVINGS · ACTIVE TIME: 15 MINUTES · TOTAL TIME: 1 HOUR

G S D

PER SERVING
(⅙ RECIPE):
Calories: 220
Calories from fat: 20
Total fat: 2 g
Saturated fat: 0 g
Trans fat: 0 g
Total carb: 39 g
Fiber: 18 g
Sugars: 10 g
Protein: 13 g
Cholesterol: 0 mg
Sodium: 800 mg
Vitamin A: 30%
Vitamin C: 10%
Calcium: 10%
Iron: 25%

Eggplant and lentils make for a kinda beefy chili that warms you to the core on a cold winter's night. If a little cocoa powder in chili is new to you, don't take my word for its deliciousness: Mexico has been rocking the chocolate and chili for thousands of years. I prefer plain old green lentils for this dish. They're easy to find and their mellow flavor works well with all the strong flavors of this recipe. Serve with Fresh Corn and Scallion Corn Bread (recipe follows), over rice, or over a baked sweet potato.

1 teaspoon olive oil
1 small onion, cut into medium dice
1 red bell pepper, cut into medium dice
3 cloves garlic, minced
1 tablespoon mild chili powder
2 teaspoons ground cumin
2 teaspoons ground coriander
2 teaspoons dried oregano
½ teaspoon ground cinnamon
¾ teaspoon salt
2 tablespoons unsweetened cocoa powder
1 cup dried green lentils, washed
4 cups vegetable broth
1 (15-ounce) can diced tomatoes
2 pounds eggplant, cut into ¾-inch cubes
2 teaspoons agave nectar or pure maple syrup
Cilantro, for garnish (optional)

TIP
For spicier chili, add ½ teaspoon of red pepper flakes when you add the garlic.

Preheat a 4-quart pot over medium-high heat. Sauté the onions and bell pepper in the oil until translucent, 5 to 7 minutes. Add the garlic and sauté for another minute, using nonstick cooking spray or a splash of water if it's sticking. Mix in the chili powder, cumin, coriander, oregano, cinnamon, and salt. Add ½ cup of the vegetable broth and the cocoa powder, and cook for about 1 more minute while stirring to dissolve the cocoa.

Add the lentils, remaining vegetable broth, diced tomatoes, and eggplant. Cover the pot and bring the mixture to a boil, keeping a close eye on it. Once it's boiling, lower the heat to a simmer and cook for about 40 minutes, until the lentils are tender and the eggplant is soft. Mix in the agave. Taste for salt and seasoning.

Let the chili sit for 10 minutes or so for maximum flavor. Serve garnished with cilantro, if you like.

∾ **NUTRITION TIP** Lentils are an amazingly nutritious little bean. So much so that those vegetarian cookbooks from the '70s seem to be all lentil dishes! Well, we're not afraid to bring this nutritional rock star into the twenty-first century. They are high in protein, iron, and fiber—all important nutrients for vegans and those who love them. One-half cup cooked lentils has 9 grams of protein, 3.2 grams of iron, 179 micrograms of folate, and 8 grams of fiber. They're also incredibly affordable—that half cup would cost you around twenty-five cents. Next time someone tells you that veganism is expensive, you answer, "Lentils." ∾

Fresh Corn & Scallion Corn Bread

SERVES 8 • ACTIVE TIME: 15 MINUTES • TOTAL TIME: 45 MINUTES

(CAN BE MADE SOY FREE IF USING NONSOY MILK)

Corn bread! The perfect accompaniment to chili. I like to cut the squares in half diagonally to form cute triangles that garnish the chili. Just because it's healthy doesn't mean it can't be adorable. Fresh corn gives this a lot of great texture and scallion makes it something to savor. Hopefully that means smaller pieces will make you satisfied, but it might mean that a loved one will have to lock up the leftovers in a safe to keep you from it.

- 1 cup unsweetened almond milk, or your preferred nondairy milk
- 1 teaspoon apple cider vinegar
- 1 cup cornmeal
- ½ cup whole wheat pastry flour or all-purpose flour
- 1 teaspoon baking powder
- ¼ teaspoon salt
- 2 tablespoons canola oil
- 2 tablespoons agave syrup or pure maple syrup
- 1 cup fresh or frozen corn kernels (thaw first if frozen)
- ½ cup finely chopped scallions

Preheat the oven to 350°F and lightly spray an 8-inch square metal baking pan with nonstick cooking spray.

In a measuring cup, wisk together the almond milk and the vinegar, and set aside to curdle.

In a large bowl, sift together the cornmeal, flour, baking powder, and salt. Create a well in the center and add the almond milk, agave, and oil. Mix just until combined. Fold in the corn and scallions.

Pour the batter into the prepared baking pan and bake for 28 to 32 minutes, until a toothpick inserted into the center comes out clean. Slice into squares and serve warm or store in an airtight container.

Quinoa, White Bean, & Kale Stew

SERVES 8 • ACTIVE TIME: 20 MINUTES • TOTAL TIME: 40 MINUTES

This is one of my winter staples, especially if I'm having a busy week, have no one to impress, and don't want to use a million dishes (big ups to the disherwasherless!). You get your beans, greens, and grains all in one pot; in this case I use white beans, kale, and quinoa. You also get about eight servings out of it, so you can either freeze it or keep it in the fridge for four days or so, having it for lunch or dinner or . . . stew for breakfast? Why not!

It's really versatile, so make up your own spice blend, use different beans and grains (although cooking time may vary for the grain), and, you know, just do whatever you want—this stew is your canvas. Prep the herb blend before proceeding with the recipe; that way you just dump everything in at the same time without much fuss.

HERB BLEND:

- ½ teaspoon fennel seeds, crushed (see tip about crushing fennel seeds, page 248)
- 1 teaspoon dried marjoram
- 1 teaspoon dried thyme
- ½ teaspoon dried rosemary
  Freshly ground black pepper

EVERYTHING ELSE:

- 1 teaspoon olive oil
- 2 cups thinly sliced leeks (white and green parts, about one average-size leek)
- 1 teaspoon salt
- 4 cloves garlic, minced
- 1 large carrot, peeled, cut into medium dice
- 1 large parsnip, peeled, cut into medium dice
- 8 cups vegetable broth

PER SERVING
(⅛ RECIPE):
Calories: 300
Calories from fat: 25
Total fat: 2.5 g
Saturated fat: 0 g
Trans fat: 0 g
Total carb: 56 g
Fiber: 9 g
Sugars: 6 g
Protein: 14 g
Cholesterol: 0 mg
Sodium: 890 mg
Vitamin A: 210%
Vitamin C: 150%
Calcium: 20%
Iron: 30%

1½ pounds Yukon Gold potatoes, cut into medium dice
1 cup dried quinoa
1 (15-ounce) can white beans, drained and rinsed
1 bunch kale (about a pound), coarse stems removed, torn into bite-size pieces

First, prepare the herb blend by stirring all its ingredients together in a small bowl.

Preheat a 4-quart pot over medium-high heat. Sauté the leeks and garlic in oil with the salt for about 3 minutes, or however long it takes you to prep your carrot and parsnip. Add the carrot and parsnip, along with the herb blend, turn up the heat to high, and sauté for a few seconds.

Add the vegetable broth, potatoes, and quinoa. Cover and bring to a boil. Once boiling, lower the heat to medium and cook for 15 minutes, until the potatoes and quinoa are tender. Add the kale and beans, and cook, stirring frequently, until the kale is wilted. Cover and simmer over low heat for 5 more minutes. Taste for salt.

When you serve this stew you may want to add a little lemon juice or a splash of balsamic vinegar or hot sauce—whatever your thing is. Or you may not!

Portobello Pepper Steak Stew

SERVES 4 • ACTIVE TIME: 30 MINUTES • TOTAL TIME: 30 MINUTES

Cooking bell peppers 'til they're slightly blackened brings them to new flavor heights. That plus red pepper flakes and black pepper makes for a really peppery and yummy stew that comes together quickly, right in your skillet. A hint of fennel seed adds a lot of interest without being overwhelming.

Portobello and seitan form a tag team of meatiness that makes this stew the perfect meal for a Super Bowl party or a particularly rough night of extreme knitting. Serve over a baked potato, or on a whole wheat roll for a sloppy sandwich. Or, for a neater sandwich, try a whole wheat pita. To get this together in 30 minutes, prep the onions and pepper while the seitan is cooking, and prep the mushrooms while the onion and peppers are cooking.

> **PER SERVING
> (¼ RECIPE):**
> Calories: 190
> Calories from fat: 35
> Total fat: 4 g
> Saturated fat: 0.5 g
> Trans fat: 0 g
> Total carb: 19 g
> Fiber: 3 g
> Sugars: 6 g
> Protein: 15 g
> Cholesterol: 0 mg
> Sodium: 740 mg
> Vitamin A: 20%
> Vitamin C: 110%
> Calcium: 6%
> Iron: 15%

- 2 teaspoons olive oil
- 2 cups seitan, sliced thinly
- 1 red onion, sliced into ¼-inch half-moons
- 1 red bell pepper, seeded and sliced in ¼-inch strips
- 1 green bell pepper, seeded and sliced in ¼-inch strips
  A big pinch of salt
- 2 portobello caps, sliced into ¼-inch strips
- 3 cloves garlic, minced
- ½ teaspoon fennel seeds, crushed (see tip)
- 1 teaspoon dried thyme
- ½ teaspoon salt
- ¼ teaspoon red pepper flakes
  Several pinches of freshly ground black pepper
- ½ cup dry red wine
- 2 cups vegetable broth
- 3 tablespoons all-purpose flour

Preheat a large, heavy-bottomed (preferably cast-iron) skillet over medium-high heat. Sauté the seitan in 1 teaspoon of the oil for about 5 minutes, until browned. Remove the seitan from the pan and set aside.

Sauté the onions and peppers and a pinch of the salt in the remaining oil until the peppers are slightly blackened, about 10 minutes. Add the mushrooms, garlic, fennel seeds, thyme, remaining salt, red pepper flakes, and black pepper, and sauté for 3 more minutes, until the mushrooms have released their moisture.

Add the red wine and bring to a boil over higher heat. The liquid should reduce in about 3 minutes.

In a measuring cup, mix the flour into the broth to dissolve into a slurry (see tip). Lower the heat a bit and add the slurry to the pan. Mix well and let thicken for a minute. Add the seitan back to the pan and let the stew thicken further; in about 5 minutes it should be slightly thickened but smooth and luscious.

Taste for salt and seasoning and serve.

> ⮑ *TIP In this recipe you're going to make what's technically called a "slurry," which means you'll be dissolving starch (flour, in this case) in liquid (broth, in this case) to use as a thickener in the stew. To get the flour dissolved quickly, pour ¼ cup of the broth in a measuring cup, then stir in the flour. When it's thick and dissolved, stir in the remaining broth. ⮐*

> ⮑ *TIP You don't need any fancy equipment to crush fennel. Sure, if you're an old hand at a mortar and pestle, then go ahead and use it. But for the rest of us, unlike many rounder seeds, fennel seed doesn't mind sitting still on a cutting board and being chopped up by a chef's knife. Carefully rock your knife back and forth over the fennel until no whole seeds are left. ⮐*

> ⮑ *TIP To get beautiful strips of bell peppers, slice them from stem to bottom. Tear out the seeds and any large pieces of the white membrane inside of the pepper. Turn them face down and slice widthwise for perfect curved strips. ⮐*

Moroccan Chickpeas & Zucchini

SERVES 6 • ACTIVE TIME: 15 MINUTES • TOTAL TIME: 1 HOUR

A fragrant, brothy, and soul-satisfying dish, with aromatic hints of cumin and cinnamon, this is a pantry staple for me. It cooks for about 45 minutes, but it's really super simple with minimal prep or fussiness. The zucchini and carrots become tender and velvety, and the slow-cooked chickpeas turn soft and comforting. Fresh mint is optional, only because this dish becomes more pantry friendly without it, but it does provide another level of flavor. Serve with whole wheat couscous, which is not gluten free.

- 1 teaspoon olive oil
- 1 smallish yellow onion, sliced thinly
- 4 cloves garlic, minced
- 1 tablespoon minced fresh ginger
- ½ teaspoon red pepper flakes
- 2 bay leaves
- 1 teaspoon ground cumin
- 1 teaspoon ground coriander
  A generous pinch of ground cinnamon
- ½ teaspoon salt
- 2 cups vegetable broth
- 1 cup baby carrots
- 2 zucchini, sliced into ¼-inch-thick half-moons
- 1 (24-ounce) can whole tomatoes
- 1 (25-ounce) can chickpeas, drained and rinsed
- 3 tablespoons chopped fresh mint, plus a little extra for garnish

Preheat a 4-quart pot over medium-high heat. Sauté the onions in the oil until translucent, about 4 minutes. Use a little nonstick cooking spray or broth if needed. Add the garlic, ginger, and red pepper flakes, and sauté for another minute.

PER SERVING (⅙ RECIPE):
Calories: 230
Calories from fat: 25
Total fat: 2.5 g
Saturated fat: 0 g
Trans fat: 0 g
Total carb: 45 g
Fiber: 10 g
Sugars: 16 g
Protein: 10 g
Cholesterol: 0 mg
Sodium: 1,010mg
Vitamin A: 110%
Vitamin C: 80%
Calcium: 15%
Iron: 20%

Add the remaining spices and salt, and sauté for about 30 seconds. Deglaze the pot with the veggie broth and mix in the carrots. Cover the pot and bring it to a boil. Once boiling, lower the heat to a simmer and cook for about 10 minutes. Add the zucchini. Break up the tomatoes with your fingers and add them to the pot, including the juice. Mix in the chickpeas.

Cover the pot and bring to a slow boil. Cook for about 15 minutes. Then adjust the lid so that there's some room for steam to escape. Cook for another 15 minutes; the liquid should reduce a bit, but not too much. Add the mint, if using, and let sit for about 10 minutes to let the flavors meld. Remove the bay leaves and taste for salt.

Serve with couscous, and garnish with mint.

Veggie Potpie Stew

SERVES 6 • ACTIVE TIME: 20 MINUTES • TOTAL TIME: 1 HOUR

The mingling of fresh thyme, carrots, and potatoes is pure comfort to me. Well, this recipe gives you permission to enjoy these timeless flavors without going through the trouble of preparing a whole potpie. Prepare the filling and enjoy it over **Caulipots** (page 54) or with sweet potato biscuits.

I usually make potpie with a roux base, which is basically flour toasted in a lot of oil or margarine. Instead, to make the gravy thick and satisfying (and lower in calories), I use a handful of yellow split peas. They up the nutrition profile considerably as well as add even more mouthwatering flavor to this stew. The stew thickens even more as it cools, so you'll need to add more water when you reheat.

PER SERVING
(⅙ RECIPE):
Calories: 230
Calories from fat: 10
Total fat: 1.5 g
Saturated fat: 0 g
Trans fat: 0 g
Total carb: 45 g
Fiber: 8 g
Sugars: 7 g
Protein: 10 g
Cholesterol: 0 mg
Sodium: 530 mg
Vitamin A: 130%
Vitamin C: 25%
Calcium: 6%
Iron: 15%

 1 teaspoon olive oil
 1 small onion, cut into medium dice
 ½ pound cremini mushrooms, sliced
 3 cloves garlic, minced
 1½ teaspoons dried sage
 ½ teaspoon salt
    Several pinches of freshly ground black pepper
 ½ cup yellow split peas
 3 cups vegetable broth
 1½ pounds russet potatoes, peeled and cut into ¾-inch chunks
 ½ pound carrots, peeled and cut into ½-inch chunks
 2 heaping tablespoons fresh thyme
 1 cup water
 ¼ cup all-purpose flour
 ¾ cup frozen peas

Preheat a 4-quart pot over medium-high heat. Sauté the onions in the oil until translucent, about 4 minutes. Add the mushrooms, garlic, sage, salt, and black pepper and sauté for 3 more minutes, until the mushrooms have released their moisture.

> ౿ TIP *Use a strong broth for this. Some sort of unchicken broth would work best!* ౿

Add the split peas and vegetable broth, cover the pot, and bring to a boil. Let boil for about 5 minutes, then add the potatoes and carrots. Lower the heat just a bit to a simmer and cook for 25 to 30 more minutes, or until the split peas are tender and the potatoes and carrots are cooked. Stir the stew occasionally to make sure it doesn't burn or stick to the bottom.

In a measuring cup, mix the flour into the water to dissolve into a slurry (see tip, page 248). Add the thyme, slurry, and frozen peas to the pan. Cook, uncovered, for about 10 more minutes, stirring often. The stew should thicken and become more and more delicious.

Taste for salt and seasoning. Serve garnished with more fresh thyme.

> **TIP** *There's a great sandwich place in NYC called S'nice, and they serve a potpie wrap. It's just what it sounds like, potpie filling in a flour wrap, and it is faboo. Try it by letting the stew cool to a manageable temperature, then wrapping a cupful up like a burrito.*

> **NUTRITION TIP** *The Pea Word: Split peas are super-duper high in protein—the half cup in this recipe adds 24 grams. Thirty percent of the calories in this recipe are from protein.*

> **TIP** *For an even creamier potpie, or if your split peas are a bit old, soak the split peas in water the night before cooking. If you prefer more texture in your split peas, then don't worry about it.*

Sweet Potato Drop Biscuits

MAKES 10 BISCUITS • ACTIVE TIME: 15 MINUTES • TOTAL TIME: 45 MINUTES

(S)

These biscuits go perfectly with the **Veggie Potpie Stew** (page 251), or anywhere a biscuit would go. Sweet potatoes not only give the biscuits a hint of sweet flavor and a pretty hue, but they also stand in for the copious amounts of shortening usually found in biscuits.

- 1 cup mashed cooked sweet potatoes
- 3 tablespoons canola oil
- 1 tablespoon pure maple syrup
- 1 teaspoon apple cider vinegar
- ½ teaspoon salt
- 1 cup all-purpose or whole wheat pastry flour, or a mix of both
- 2 teaspoons baking powder
- 1 teaspoon ground nutmeg
- 2 to 3 tablespoons cold water

PER SERVING
(1 BISCUIT):
Calories: 100
Calories from fat: 40
Total fat: 4.5 g
Saturated fat: 0 g
Trans fat: 0 g
Total carb: 15 g
Fiber: 2 g
Sugars: 3 g
Protein: 2 g
Cholesterol: 0 mg
Sodium: 125 mg
Vitamin A: 80%
Vitamin C: 6%
Calcium: 6%
Iron: 4%

Preheat the oven to 400°F and cover a baking sheet with parchment paper.

In a medium-size bowl, mix together the mashed sweet potatoes, oil, maple syrup, apple cider vinegar, and salt. Use a sifter to sift in the flour, baking powder, and nutmeg.

Fold the flour into the sweet potato mixture with a wooden spoon until the dry ingredients are moistened and crumbly; be careful not to over-mix. Add 2 tablespoons water and lightly knead five or six times until the dough holds together, adding the extra water if needed. Don't knead too much or it will toughen the biscuits.

Drop the dough in golf ball–size pieces onto the prepared baking sheet. Bake for 12 to 15 minutes, or until the tops are lightly browned and firm to the touch.

> ∿ TIP To make mashed sweet potatoes, preheat the oven to 400°F. Place the sweet potatoes in the oven and bake until done. I think it takes ½ pound to make 1 cup of mashed sweet potatoes. What I would do is bake a few for dinner the night before and then reserve the extras to make these biscuits within one or two nights. ∿

Smoky Tempeh & Greens Stew

SERVES 6 • ACTIVE TIME: 15 MINUTES • TOTAL TIME: ABOUT 45 MINUTES

A filling, stick-to-your-ribs tomato stew with succulent bites of tempeh and earthy greens. The smokiness comes from smoked paprika, which is readily available in the spice section of most supermarkets these days. It's a fabulous spice to have in your arsenal because it adds tons of flavor without adding any fat or sugar. This recipe is a wonderful showcase for building flavor and texture instead of just pouring in the oil.

Eat this stew straight up or ladled over basmati rice. Chop all your veggies while the tempeh is cooking and you'll have this stew going in no time.

2 teaspoons oil

8 ounces tempeh, torn into bite-size pieces

1 medium-size yellow onion, diced finely

2 bay leaves

2 teaspoons dried thyme
Freshly ground black pepper

1 cup baby carrots, sliced in half lengthwise

1 bunch (about a pound) kale, chard, or other leafy greens, stems chopped separately (see tip about stems) and leaves chopped roughly

4 cloves garlic, minced

¼ cup dry red wine or water

1½ teaspoons salt

1 (28-ounce) can crushed tomatoes

1 cup vegetable broth

4 teaspoons smoked paprika

1 cup frozen baby lima beans

Preheat a 5- to 6-quart, heavy-bottomed pot (see tip) over medium-high heat. Sauté the tempeh in 1 teaspoon of the oil for about 10 minutes, until lightly browned. Remove the tempeh from the pot and set aside.

In the same pot, sauté the onion, bay leaves, thyme, and several pinches of pepper in the remaining teaspoon of oil for about 3 minutes. Add the carrots and the stems from the greens. Partially cover and cook for about 10 minutes, stirring often, to soften the carrots.

Add the garlic and sauté for about a minute. Deglaze the pan with red wine. Mix in the salt, crushed tomatoes, water, and paprika. Cover and bring to a simmer. Add the greens, cover, and cook for about 10 minutes, stirring often, until the greens are completely cooked down. Add the lima beans and return the tempeh to the pot, then turn off the heat. Taste and adjust for salt and seasonings.

Let the stew sit for 10 minutes, uncovered, until the lima beans are heated through. Remove the bay leaves and serve.

TIP I like to use a wide 5- or 6-quart pot for this dish. When you're sautéing tempeh in the minimum amount of oil, the more surface area, the better. If you don't have such a big pot, it's best to use a skillet and then proceed with the rest of the recipe in your smaller 4-quart pot.

NOTE If you don't like or don't have tempeh, use a 15-ounce can of white beans instead. This will also shave 10 minutes off your cooking time, and save you a teaspoon of oil. Add the beans at the end along with the lima beans.

TIP You can and should use the stems from the greens in stews. They add great texture and bulk, not to mention that fiber we all love so much. Just chop them thinly and add them when you add the carrots.

Kidney Bean & Butternut Jamba Stew

SERVES 4 • ACTIVE TIME: 20 MINUTES • TOTAL TIME: 40 MINUTES

This stew is inspired by jambalaya, only it's a whole lot more saucy. When I think kidney beans, I think, "This is a bean's bean." Big, meaty, and substantial, it demands to be front and center, not mashed or pureed.

The slight sweetness of butternut squash is a natural partner in this spicy stew with its Creole seasonings. I use white basmati here because of its shorter cooking time. If you'd like to use brown, then add the squash about 20 minutes after you add the rice and tack on about 20 more minutes' cooking time. Everything can come together quickly if you prep the squash while the onion and other veggies are sautéing. (See butternut squash tip, page 80.)

1 teaspoon olive oil
1 smallish yellow onion, diced small
1 green bell pepper, seeded and diced small
2 ribs celery, sliced thinly
4 cloves garlic, minced
2 bay leaves
2 teaspoons paprika
½ teaspoon cayenne
1 teaspoon dried thyme
1 teaspoon dried oregano
1 teaspoon salt
2 cups vegetable broth
1 (28-ounce) can whole tomatoes
1½ pounds butternut squash, cut into ¾-inch chunks
½ cup white basmati rice
1 (15-ounce) can kidney beans, drained and rinsed

Preheat a 4-quart pot over medium-high heat. Sauté the onion, pepper, celery, and garlic in the oil with a pinch of salt for about 7 minutes. Use a little nonstick cooking spray or broth if things are sticking.

Add the bay leaves, spices, herbs, and remaining salt, and sauté for about 30 seconds. Add the veggie broth and tomatoes. Use a potato masher to mash up the tomatoes. Add the butternut squash, rice, and kidney beans. Cover the pot and bring to a boil. Once boiling, lower the heat to a simmer and cook the stew for about 20 minutes, until the butternut squash is tender and the rice is cooked.

Remove the bay leaves, taste for salt, and serve.

> ∾ NUTRITION TIP
>
> *Squash and its relatives are magnificent holders of nutrients. They can be stored long after harvest without losing significant amounts, which is a requirement for those in colder climates who are trying to eat local and are limiting fruits and vegetables shipped from afar.* ∾

Irish Stew with Potatoes & Seitan

SERVES 4 • ACTIVE TIME: 15 MINUTES • TOTAL TIME: 45 MINUTES

Dear Ireland: I know you eat more than beer and potatoes! Love, Isa. That said . . . I love cooking with beer and potatoes and I imagine myself in the pub from *The Wicker Man* whenever I eat a bowlful. The original, of course, not the Nicholas Cage remake. Beer adds great depth of flavor, and a splash of lemon juice at the end brightens everything up. Serve with a hunk of good bread. Like the **Portobello Pepper Steak Stew** (page 247), this comes together right in your skillet. It requires a lid, but if you don't have a large lid just use a cookie sheet to cover the pan.

2	teaspoons olive oil
2	cups seitan, sliced thinly
1	small onion, quartered and sliced thinly
½	teaspoon salt
3	cloves garlic, minced
	Freshly ground black pepper
1	teaspoon dried thyme
2	bay leaves
1	cup good beer, preferably ale
1¼	pounds Yukon Gold potatoes (2 average-size), cut into ¾-inch chunks
½	pound carrots, sliced diagonally into pieces ½-inch thick
3½	cups broth
1	tablespoon tomato paste
3	tablespoons all-purpose flour
¼	pound green beans, ends trimmed, cut into inch-long pieces (1 cup)
2	tablespoons freshly squeezed lemon juice

Preheat a large, heavy-bottomed (preferably cast-iron) skillet over medium-high heat. Sauté the seitan in 1 teaspoon of the oil for about 5 minutes, until browned. This is a good time to prep everything else. Remove the seitan from the pan and set aside.

In the same pan, sauté the onions and a pinch of the salt in the remaining oil until translucent, 4 to 7 minutes. Add the garlic, pepper, thyme, and bay leaves, and sauté for about a minute, until the garlic is fragrant.

Add the beer and remaining salt and turn up the heat to bring to a boil. The liquid should reduce in about 3 minutes.

Add the potatoes and carrots along with 2 cups of the vegetable broth. Cover and bring to a boil. Once boiling, add the green beans and lower the heat to bring to a simmer. Simmer for about 15 minutes, or until the potatoes are fork tender. Mix in the tomato paste.

In a measuring cup, mix the flour into the remaining broth to dissolve into a slurry (see tip, page 248). Lower the heat a bit and add the slurry to the pan. Mix well and let thicken for a minute. Add the seitan back to the pan along with the lemon juice and let thicken further; in about 5 minutes it should be perfectly thick but still smooth. Taste for salt and seasonings, and serve!

Eggplant Provençal

SERVES 6 • ACTIVE TIME: 20 MINUTES • TOTAL TIME: 40 MINUTES

Of all the styles of cooking, the one most foreign to me is French. I've heard that a vegan can eat extraordinarily well in France, and I'm not surprised, but if you thumb through a French cookbook you will mostly see recipes that require pounds of butter, pints of cream, and other unspeakable horrors. So I'd always shied away from it. But I recently got a cookbook of Provençal cooking, referring to the Provence area of France, and the recipes were instantly appealing. Olives, fennel, tomato . . . it's a vegan's dream! Swap out some of those meats for lentils and super meaty eggplant and you've got yourself a winner of a stew. Serve over rice or with a big hunk of bread.

1	teaspoon olive oil
1	small onion, sliced thinly
1	baseball-size fennel bulb, sliced thinly
3	cloves garlic, minced
	A pinch of salt
	Freshly ground black pepper
2	bay leaves
1¼	pounds eggplant, cut into ¾-inch chunks
1¼	pounds Yukon Gold potatoes, cut into ¾-inch chunks (2 average-size potatoes)
½	pound carrots, sliced diagonally into ½-inch-thick pieces
½	cup dried red lentils
2	teaspoons dried thyme
1	teaspoon dried marjoram
¾	cup dry red wine
2	cups vegetable broth
½	cup finely chopped kalamata olives
1	(6-ounce) can tomato sauce

Preheat a 4-quart pot over medium-high heat. Sauté the onion, fennel, and garlic in the oil with a pinch of salt, for about 7 minutes. Use a little nonstick cooking spray or water if things are sticking.

Add the remaining salt, pepper, and bay leaves, and sauté for about 30 seconds. Mix in the eggplant, potatoes, carrots, red lentils, thyme, and marjoram. Add the wine and veggie broth. The liquid should just about cover everything, but it's okay if some vegetables are poking out; they will cook down.

Cover and bring to a boil, then lower to a simmer. Cook for about 20 minutes, until the potatoes are fork tender and the eggplant is mostly broken down. The lentils should be soft as well, but depending on your lentils it may take 10 or so more minutes.

Mix in the olives and tomato sauce and cook for 5 more minutes to get the flavors melded.

Remove the bay leaves, taste for salt, and serve.

Surefire Seitan

MAKES 1 POUND; SERVES 4 • ACTIVE TIME: 10 MINUTES • TOTAL TIME: 1 HOUR

Seitan can get pretty expensive, even in small quantities. Simmering your own seitan from vital wheat gluten flour is not only more cost effective, but it's more delicious effective, too! And it really isn't very hard. If you've ever mixed up any dough, seitan-making isn't any different. It's just a small matter of a little kneading and then plopping into a simmering broth. So make the initial investment of a bag of the flour, and then seitan will be yours for weeks to come!

BROTH:

8 cups vegetable broth (the powdered or bouillon kind works great)
¼ cup soy sauce

SEITAN:

1 cup vital wheat gluten flour
3 tablespoons chickpea flour
½ cup cold vegetable broth
¼ cup soy sauce
1 tablespoon freshly squeezed lemon juice
2 teaspoons olive oil
2 cloves garlic, pressed or grated on a Microplane grater

Begin the broth: Bring the 8 cups of vegetable broth and ¼ cup of soy sauce to a boil in a covered 4-quart stockpot. Meanwhile, prepare the seitan.

In a large bowl, mix together the gluten and chickpea flour. Make a well in the center and add the ½ cup of cold broth, the ¼ cup of soy sauce, and the lemon juice, olive oil, and garlic. Mix with a wooden spoon until most of the moisture has been absorbed and has partially clumped up with the dry ingredients. Use your hands to knead for about 3 minutes, until it's an elastic dough. Divide into four equal pieces with a knife and then knead those individual pieces in your hand just to stretch them out a bit. Let rest until the broth is ready.

Once the broth has boiled, lower the heat to a simmer. It should be bubbling, but not very rapidly. I use moderate low heat. Drop in the gluten pieces and partially cover the pot so that a little steam can escape. Simmer for about 45 minutes, then turn off the heat and let sit for 15 more minutes.

Remove the seitan from the broth and place it in a strainer until it is cool enough to handle.

The Elements of a Bowl

ANYONE WHO HAS BEEN VEGETARIAN FOR ANY AMOUNT OF time, or anyone who has ever stepped foot into a '90s health food restaurant, for that matter, will be familiar with "The Bowl"—an upside-down hard hat filled with some combination of veggies, grains, and beans plus a sauce or two. It might not sound like much but when done up at home, bowls can be lifesavers—delicious, delicious lifesavers. Take them to lunch, have the ingredients waiting at home in the fridge to throw together, or just make all the components on the spot. As a rule, bowls don't have to be complicated.

Typically my bowls consist of a sauce, a grain, a bean, and a green. Sometimes tempeh or tofu is the bean, or sometimes when you're super hungry, you can throw caution to the wind and have beans *and* tofu. The real beauty of the bowl is that you can eat the same thing for a month, a year, the rest of your life! And yet never have to eat the same thing again. Call it Isa's Paradox.

The grain: Quinoa is a favorite because it cooks so fast. Brown basmati rice is a close second when I've got a little more time. Not really a grain, but buckwheat soba is an occasional treat. Occasional only, because it's a bit more pricy than my old standbys. I love whole wheat couscous, but it tends to not be as versatile; I usually have to limit it to Middle Eastern or Mediterranean flavors. And if I'm feeling irreverent I'll get crazy with kasha, millet, or barley.

A good tip when rocking the bowl on a weeknight is to put on your grain to cook the instant you walk through the door. Don't even take your jacket off! Don't even pet your cat! If your significant other tries to kiss you hello, push him or her aside and get thee to the kitchen. Once the grain is going, you have some breathing room to settle in and relax, then prep all the other additions to your bowl.

The bean: Well, I'm a chickpea girl through and through, so my little garbanzo angels get the most play. But I do vary my bean. Popular favorites are: black-eyed peas, pinto beans, black beans, azuki beans, du Puy lentils, kidney beans, and cannellini beans. The canned-or-homemade question? That's really up to you. When I am not creating a bean dish per se; rather, just eating them in all their minimalist glory, I prefer to simmer my own beans. There's nothing more nurturing than a pot of beans simmering on the stove top. But that isn't always possible or practical, so oftentimes, when I come through the door famished, I rinse off some beans and throw them in the mix. If the rest of the food is warm, the beans don't necessarily need to be. But if you do want to warm them up, toss them into the steamer for a minute or two after you steam your veggies.

The veggie: Refer to the steamer info in the veggie chapter (page 85). Steaming just makes the most sense for a bowl. Really, the flavor is coming from the sauce, so keep everything as simple as possible.

The sauce: This is the fun part! I try to have sauces or dressings prepped in advance. Because the recipes in this book are so healthy and low in fat and calories, with many of them you can use a double serving if you like things super saucy. Some of my favorite all-around sauces are Green Goddess Garlic Dressing, Sanctuary Dressing, Silky Chickpea Gravy, Carrot-Ginger Dressing, and Caesar Chavez Dressing.

Then there's the actual bowl. Can you eat your bowl on a plate? No! Well, maybe. But part of the fun of bowls is the actual bowl. It's a casual meal, so pick oversize bowls that you can fit on your lap or take outside to eat on the porch or fire escape. They should have plenty of space for filling with veggies and tossing around your ingredients as you see fit. I love ceramic bowls, either vintage ones or yuppy ones from Crate and Barrel.

Fill your bowl to the brim and it will spill. Keep sharpening your knife and it will blunt.
—*Lao Tzu*

BOWLS TO GO

Because all of the ingredients taste great at room temperature, bowls make an excellent lunch to go. You can either pack all the elements bento box style, in individual compartments, or just place everything but the sauce in Tupperware. The sauce, of course, will go in a little container. If you store your lunch in the fridge, take it out about an hour before you're ready to eat, just to get the chill off it. Mix together, pour the sauce on, and bon appétit!

Mexicana Kale Bowl
Brown rice, black beans, steamed kale, steamed sweet potato, **Red Velvet Mole** (page 134), chopped fresh cilantro

Supergreen Bowl
Quinoa, steamed kale and broccoli, edamame,

Green Goddess Garlic Dressing (page 26), chopped fresh parsley and chives

Peanut-Lime Tempeh Bowl
Quinoa, steamed broccoli, sauteed tempeh, **Peanut–Lime Dragon Dressing** (page 34)

Nori Bowl
Brown rice, steamed broccoli, azuki beans, **Carrot–Ginger Dressing** (page 52), shredded nori.

Mediterranean Bowl
Bulgur, roasted cauliflower, chickpeas, **Caesar Chavez Dressing** (page 43)

Romesco Bowl
Quinoa, white beans, grilled zucchini, **Romesco Dressing** (page 47)

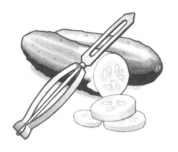

Vegan Bowl
All the bowls are vegan of course, but this one is especially so: brown rice, baked tofu, steamed kale, **Caesar Chavez Dressing** (page 43)

Soba Bowl
Soba noodles, steamed broccoli and zucchini, black beans, **Green Onion–Miso Vinaigrette** (page 21)

Gravy Bowl
Brown rice, baked tempeh, steamed kale, and **Silky Chickpea Gravy** (page 56)

The Importance of Eating Sandwich

SANDWICHES & WRAPS

OR THE ANTIFORK SET. I DON'T THINK I REALLY NEED TO TOUT the benefits of handheld food, do I? This section is great for ideas on what to do with leftovers, or for those times when you want to drag a loved one to the park and have a picnic.

Sandwiches get a bad rap for diets, but if you use the right ingredients they can fit right into your lifestyle. The solution to unhealthy, dream-crushing sandwiches are whole-grain breads; the luscious sauces and dressings from this here book, instead of crazy–holy cow 14 grams of fat in one tablespoon of mayo; lots of fresh veggies; and a little ingenuity.

For the wraps, we choose 12-inch whole wheat tortillas, but there are many gluten free options out there, too. Wraps taste best when they've been warmed up just a tad, because they can be kind of stiff coming out of the fridge. It isn't mandatory, but if you've got the time, microwave or steam your wrap for about 30 seconds before assembling.

How to wrap with authority:

Breakfast Sandwich

A classic! Eat this baby on the run. You'll look cool carrying it and you'll keep yourself full until lunchtime.

Toasted whole wheat English muffin spread with 2 tablespoons **Caesar Chavez Dressing** (page 43), 1/3 cup **Curry Scrambled Tofu with Wilted Arugula** (page 156), topped with four strips **Eggplant Bacon** (page 42).

Cashew Miso Mayo

MAKES 8 TABLESPOONS • ACTIVE TIME: 7 MINUTES • TOTAL COOKING TIME: 7 MINUTES

If you're looking for something creamy to spread onto your sandwiches then you've come to the right place. I take my mayo seriously, and this has all but completely replaced store-bought vegan mayonnaise for me, so you know I am not messing around. I'll still keep some store-bought in the fridge for special potato salad occasions, but really, at over 10 grams of fat per tablespoon, what's the point? Note though, this is cashew miso mayo, and although it's thoroughly scrumptious it doesn't taste exactly like mayo, so it's great for replacing it in things like sandwiches and salads, but don't expect it to taste exactly the same. Do expect creaminess from the cashews, depth of flavor from the miso and tanginess from apple cider vinegar. And also expect killer BLTs.

NOTE: To make it easier to get the mayo smooth, soak the cashews in water for at least an hour. Then drain and they're ready to use.

- ¼ cup raw cashews
- ¼ cup red miso
- ¼ cup water
- 1 tablespoon apple cider vinegar

Place everything in a small food processor and blend like the dickens. If you only have a large food processor, consider doubling the recipe so that you get the volume you need to really get this whipped up good. Depending on your processor, it might take up to 5 minutes to really get the cashews smooth.

PER SERVING (1 TABLESPOON):

Calories: 35	Total carb: 4 g	Sodium: 125 mg
Calories from fat: 20	Fiber: 0 g	Vitamin A: 0%
Total fat: 2 g	Sugars: 2 g	Vitamin C: 0%
Saturated fat: 0 g	Protein: 1 g	Calcium: 0%
Trans fat: 0 g	Cholesterol: 0 mg	Iron: 0%

Buffalo Wrap

Hot and spicy tempeh is tempered by cool and creamy coleslaw. You don't have to be in a sports bar to eat this, but for the first time in your life, they wouldn't laugh you out of there. On second thought, they probably would.

½ cup **Buffalo Tempeh** (page 161), ¾ cup **Cool Slaw** (page 38) in a wrap.

Hummus Among Us Wrap

Yes, I eat hummus every day. Yes, it's embarrassing. Now you have a discreet wrap in which you can eat your hummus in peace, away from the world's harsh glaring judgmental eye.

⅓ cup **Hummus** (page 137), any variation, wrapped up with ½ cup chopped romaine lettuce, drizzled with 2 tablespoons **Balsamic Vinaigrette** (page 17), sliced tomato, cucumber, and red onion.

Open-Faced Portobello Reuben

A Jewish deli staple; if you're a fan of tangy, juicy, and messy on rye, then the Reuben is for you.

Grilled Portobellos (page 103) on one slice toasted rye bread, spread with 2 tablespoons **Caesar Chavez Dressing** (page 43) and 1 teaspoon ketchup, topped with ¼ cup sauerkraut, served with a pickle on the side.

The Moskowitz Club Wrap

The Moskowitz Club is an elite place where you get to eat absolutely everything you've ever wanted in one wrap.

Wrap up four pieces **Baked Tofu** (page 144), 6 pieces **Eggplant Bacon** (page 42), ½ cup chopped romaine lettuce, ¼ cup sprouts, ¼ cup shredded lettuce, sliced red onions, sliced pickles, and 2 tablespoons **Cashew–Miso Mayo** (see sidebar).

Caesar Chavez Wrap

I can't get enough of Caesar salad; we are in a completely codependent relationship. Having a way to take it with me only makes things worse.

Toss together 1 cup romaine lettuce with ¼ cup sautéed **Surefire Seitan** (page 262), 2 tablespoons sliced black olives, and 3 tablespoons **Caesar Chavez Dressing** (page 43). Wrap up in whole wheat wrap.

Bee Ell Tees

This sandwich makes me feel like I'm sitting in a luncheonette, on one of those stools at the counter that you would spin around on as a kid until you got dizzy and fell off and broke something and had to be taken to the hospital. Or maybe it just makes me feel like I'm eating a really satisfying BLT!

For the bread you can use two slices whole wheat bread, or two slices of a thin whole wheat bun, sometimes called a sandwich thin (they only have 100 calories), or for even less calories, ½ a whole wheat pita (that comes in at 60 calories). 1 tablespoon **Cashew-Miso Mayo** (see sidebar) on each slice, layered with romaine lettuce, six slices **Eggplant Bacon** (page 42), and a slice of tomato.

Thanksgiving Leftovers Wrap

I got this idea from my favoritest vegetarian sandwich shop, S'nice, in NYC. You can eat it warm, but it's also perfectly delicious at room temperature.

1 cup **Veggie Potpie Stew** (page 251), ¼ cup cranberry sauce, rolled up in a wrap.

Falafel Wrap

This makes perfect sense, because many falafel houses do serve their falafels as wraps. The Green Goddess Garlic Dressing is a nice touch for its hint of tahini, but it's not totally necessary if you don't have any prepared.

4 **Falafel** patties (page 121), ¼ cup any variatation **Hummus** (page 137), ½ cup shredded lettuce, ¼ cup chopped tomato, sliced red onion. Optional: ¼ cup **Green Goddess Garlic Dressing** (page 26).

Wrapper's Delight

If you check out the prepared foods in the deli case at Whole Foods Market, you'll see that anything and everything can be thrown into a wrap and they'll charge you $5.99 for the pleasure! So don't be afraid to wrap things that seem unconventional to you; convention has to start somewhere. Many of the stews in this book translate perfectly into wraps; just make sure that they are cold or at room temperature when you wrap them, so that they're good and thick.

Some suggestions:

2nd Ave. Vegetable Korma (page 226)
Curried Chickpeas & Greens (page 228)
Classic Black Bean & Veggie Chili (page 236)
Portobello Pepper Steak Stew (page 247)
Moroccan Chickpeas & Zucchini (page 249)
Kidney Bean and Butternut Jamba Stew
   (page 256)

Taco Night

Tacos are sneaky little guys. They seem kind of decadent and potentially greasy, but really, what you've got here is lots of scrumptious and satisfying whole foods: some healthy corn tortillas, fresh veggies, and legumes. They're also perfect for entertaining, because everyone can take as much as they want; no need to go overboard just because everyone else is. And hey, if you do decide it's a night for going overboard, tacos are not a bad way to do it.

Must-haves for Taco Night:
Corn tortillas
Shredded lettuce
Guacamame (page 23)
Unfried Refried Beans (page 136)
Chili-Lime-Rubbed Tofu (page 155)
Portobello Chimichurri (page 104)
Steamed Plantains (page 129)
Fresh Tomato Salsa Dressing (page 23)

Potato Toppings

What could be simpler than baking a potato, splitting it in two, topping it off, and calling it dinner? Baked potatoes make so much sense when you're looking for low fat, filling, and easy. And, come on, who doesn't love a potato? You can really become a potato artist by combining different sauces, veggies, and beans to top off your taters.

To bake russet potatoes, preheat the oven to 350°F, scrub the potatoes clean, poke with a fork a dozen times, and wrap with tin foil. An average-size potato takes about an hour in the oven. Bake a bunch of potatoes at the beginning of the week and keep them on hand to reheat.

Some of my favorite potato toppings are:
Steamed broccoli, **Easy Breezy Cheezy Sauce**
   (page 173), and **Eggplant Bacon** (page 42)
Surefire Seitan (page 262), **Sautéed Kale** (page
   89) and **Silky Chickpea Gravy** (page 56)
Roasted Cauliflower (page 179) and **Sanctuary Dressing** (page 29)
Black Beans, sautéed spinach, and **Red Velvet Mole** (page 134).
Buffalo Tempeh (page 161), **Caesar Chavez Dressing** (page 43), and grilled zucchini.

ACKNOWLEDGMENTS

Thank you to my assistants throughout the book!
Jenny "Hot Rod" Hinshaw, for slicing, dicing (and watching the kitties!)
Lauren Fitzgerald for her amazing palate and knife skills
Amy Gedgaudas for cooking her weight in curry

Also a special thanks to
Seth Wood for the beautiful cover art and illustrations.
Clara Ridabock for help with the Paprikas photo
Virgnia Payne for cooking a ton for the food photos
Lexa Walsh, for being a great neighbor and making lots of yucca
Kittee Berns for cooking for some food photos, love you!

And as always, thanks to my agent Marc Gerald and the Agency Group, my publisher Katie McHugh at Perseus and production manager Christine Marra.

For this cookbook, testers really needed to give their all. It wasn't enough to know that a recipe worked and tasted good, but since this book was all about diet and healthiness, testers had to go above and beyond. Did it keep them full? How was the portion size? Did it work with their diet plan? Testers were so diligent in their answering of these questions and so helpful with their feedback. This book would be nothing without them! Thank you guys!

Lucy Allbaugh
Michelle Citrin
Raelene Coburn
Allicia Cormier
Mike Crooker & Liz Bujack
Jess DeNoto
Tiffaney Dugan
Megan Duke
Chris Duvall
Melisser Elliott
Ryan Full
Paula Gross
Cara Heberling
Eryn Hiscock
Anna Hood
Teressa Jackson

Fay Kahn
Angelina Kelly
Carla Kelly
Jocelyn Kimmel
Jenny Kopanic
Kim Lahn
Megan McClellan
Jennifer McVea
Rachel Lawrence Middleton
Allison Nordahl
Rebecca Padrick
Thalia C. Palmer
Carol Perryman
Patrizia Pipitone
Stephanie Roy
Dayna Rozental

Luciana Rushing
Amanda Sacco
Rosemary Savoia
Rebecca Schaffer
Molly Tanzer
Megan Smythe Todd
Jackie Topol
Theresa Victor
Claudia Weber
Shanell Dawn Williams
Kirstin Wilson
Mat Winser
Angela White
Danielle Leda White
Liz Wyman

APPENDIX: RECIPES BY ICON

ⓖ GLUTEN FREE RECIPES

Full-On Salads

Totally Stuffed Sides

Rub-Your-Tummy Veggies

Main Event Beans

Sink-Your-Teeth-Into Tofu & Tempeh

Talk Pasta to Me (& Noodles!)

Talk Pasta to Me (& Noodles!)

Soul-Satisfying Soups

Comfort Curries, Chilies, & Stews

INDEX

ABOUT THE AUTHORS

ISA CHANDRA MOSKOWITZ

Isa Chandra Moskowitz is an award-winning vegan chef and author of several best-selling cookbooks, including *Veganomicon*, *Vegan with a Vengeance*, *Vegan Cupcakes Take Over the World*, *Vegan Brunch*, and *Vegan Cookies Invade Your Cookie Jar*. A Brooklyn native who began her vegan cooking journey more than twenty years ago, she is inspired by New York City's diverse cuisine. She has been featured in many print and online publications including *Saveur*, *The New York Times*, *The Washington Post*, *VegNews*, *Herbivore*, *Bust*, and more, as well as on NPR and Portland's *AM Northwest*. You can find her cooking and writing at The Post Punk Kitchen (theppk.com).

MATTHEW RUSCIGNO, MPH, RD

Matt Ruscigno completed his Master's Degree in Public Health and certification as a Registered Dietitian at Loma Linda University, one of only a handful of professionally-accredited schools promoting vegetarian nutrition. He is active with the American Dietetic Association's Vegetarian Nutrition Dietary Practice Group. Passionate about social justice, Matt educates low-income students about nutrition with the Network for a Healthy California and teaches community college in South Central Los Angeles. Matt also advises vegan athletes on ways to maximize their performance during training and events. He has participated in numerous ultra-endurance bicycle and triathlon events throughout the world.